Francis K.O. Yuen, DSW, ACSW
Editor

International Perspectives on Disability Services: The Same But Different

International Perspectives on Disability Services: The Same But Different has been co-published simultaneously as *Journal of Social Work in Disability & Rehabilitation*, Volume 2, Numbers 2/3 2003.

Pre-publication
REVIEWS,
COMMENTARIES,
EVALUATIONS . . .

"**O**F VALUE TO THOSE PROVIDING DIRECT SERVICE TO PEOPLE WITH DISABILITIES AS WELL AS THOSE WHO DESIGN AND ADMINISTER PROGRAMS. Examines disability issues from an international perspective. . . . Readers will learn how people with disabilities in other countries adapt to their status as a minority group. SERVICE PROVIDERS IN THE DISABILITY FIELD WILL BENEFIT FROM READING THIS BOOK if they wish to enrich their practice."

Roland Meinert, PhD
President, Missouri Association for Social Welfare

"**O**ne of the first principles student social workers are taught is that they should not be judgmental. Some of the authors of the writings in this book go further. They invite readers to see the world from the viewpoint of disabled people. It is a very different perspective. Instead of using social work skills to enable disabled people to adapt to a hostile environment and society, why not change the society so the barriers to their full inclusion are removed? The services offered to disabled people often say far more about the mindset of the provider than about the disabled person. THIS BOOK EXPLAINS THIS VALUABLE LESSON."

Bert Massie, CBE, BA(Hons), CQSW,
Chairman
Disability Rights Commission
Great Britain
formerly Chief Executive
The Royal Association for Disability and Rehabilitation (RADAR), London, England

"**U**NIQUE. . . . In eight EXCEPTIONAL AND WELL-DOCUMENTED chapters, Yuen and his co-authors touch on a range of urgent concerns in presenting international perspectives on the disabled and the services they are (and are not) offered. . . . Cross-cultural components are given illuminating attention."

Professor John L. Erlich
Division of Social Work
California State University
Sacramento

The Haworth Social Work Practice Press
An Imprint of The Haworth Press, Inc.

New York • London • Victoria (AU)
www.HaworthPress.com

International Perspectives on Disability Services: The Same But Different

International Perspectives on Disability Services: The Same But Different has been co-published simultaneously as *Journal of Social Work in Disability & Rehabilitation*, Volume 2, Numbers 2/3 2003.

The *Journal of Social Work in Disability & Rehabilitation* Monographic "Separates"

Below is a list of "separates," which in serials librarianship means a special issue simultaneously published as a special journal issue or double-issue *and* as a "separate" hardbound monograph. (This is a format which we also call a "DocuSerial.")

"Separates" are published because specialized libraries or professionals may wish to purchase a specific thematic issue by itself in a format which can be separately cataloged and shelved, as opposed to purchasing the journal on an on-going basis. Faculty members may also more easily consider a "separate" for classroom adoption.

"Separates" are carefully classified separately with the major book jobbers so that the journal tie-in can be noted on new book order slips to avoid duplicate purchasing.

You may wish to visit Haworth's website at . . .

http://www.HaworthPress.com

. . . to search our online catalog for complete tables of contents of these separates and related publications.

You may also call 1-800-HAWORTH (outside US/Canada: 607-722-5857), or Fax 1-800-895-0582 (outside US/Canada: 607-771-0012), or e-mail at:

docdelivery@haworthpress.com

International Perspectives on Disability Services: The Same But Different, edited by Francis K. O. Yuen, DSW (Vol. 2, No. 2/3, 2003). *"One of the first principles student social workers are taught is that they should not be judgmental. Some of the authors of the writings in this book go further. They invite readers to see the world from the viewpoint of disabled people. It is a very different perspective. Instead of using social work skills to enable disabled people to adapt to a hostile environment and society, why not change the society so the barriers to their full inclusion are removed? The services offered to disabled people often say far more about the mindset of the provider than about the disabled person. This book explains this valuable lesson." (Bert Massie, CBE, BA(Hons), CQSW, Chairman, Disability Rights Commission, Great Britain; formerly Chief Executive, The Royal Association for Disability and Rehabilitation (RADAR), London, England)*

International Perspectives on Disability Services: The Same But Different

Francis K. O. Yuen
Editor

International Perspectives on Disability Services: The Same But Different has been co-published simultaneously as *Journal of Social Work in Disability & Rehabilitation*, Volume 2, Numbers 2/3 2003.

THSWPP

The Haworth Social Work Practice Press
An Imprint of The Haworth Press, Inc.

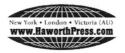

New York • London • Victoria (AU)
www.HaworthPress.com

Published by

Haworth Social Work Practice Press®, 10 Alice Street, Binghamton, NY 13904-1580 USA

Haworth Social Work Practice Press® is an imprint of The Haworth Press, Inc., 10 Alice Street, Binghamton, NY 13904-1580 USA.

International Perspectives on Disability Services: The Same But Different has been co-published simultaneously as *Journal of Social Work in Disability & Rehabilitation*, Volume 2, Numbers 2/3 2003.

The development, preparation, and publication of this work has been undertaken with great care. However, the publisher, employees, editors, and agents of The Haworth Press and all imprints of The Haworth Press, Inc., including The Haworth Medical Press® and Pharmaceutical Products Press®, are not responsible for any errors contained herein or for consequences that may ensue from use of materials or information contained in this work. Opinions expressed by the author(s) are not necessarily those of The Haworth Press, Inc.

Cover design by Lora Wiggins.

Library of Congress Cataloging-in-Publication Data

International perspectives on disability services : the same but different / Francis K.O. Yuen, Editor.
    p. cm.
    Co-published simultaneously as Journal of social work in disability & rehabilitation, Volume 2, Number 2/3 2003.
    Includes bibliographical references and index.
    ISBN 0-7890-2092-0 (hard cover : alk. paper) – ISBN 0-7890-2093-9 (soft cover : alk. paper)
    1. People with disabilities–Services for–Cross-cultural studies. I. Yuen, Francis K.O. II. Journal of social work in disability & rehabilitation.

HV1568.I597 2004
362.4–dc22   ·   2003024503

Indexing, Abstracting & Website/Internet Coverage

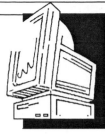

This section provides you with a list of major indexing & abstracting services. That is to say, each service began covering this periodical during the year noted in the right column. Most Websites which are listed below have indicated that they will either post, disseminate, compile, archive, cite or alert their own Website users with research-based content from this work. (This list is as current as the copyright date of this publication.)

Abstracting, Website/Indexing Coverage . . . . Year When Coverage Began

- *CNPIEC Reference Guide: Chinese National Directory of Foreign Periodicals* **2002**

- *Educational Research Abstracts (ERA) (online database)* <http://www.tandf.co.uk/era> **2002**

- *e-psyche, LLC <http://www.e-psyche.net>* **2002**

- *Exceptional Child Education Resources (ECER), (CD/ROM from SilverPlatter and hard copy)* <http://www.ericec.org/ecer-db.html> **2002**

- *Family & Society Studies Worldwide <http://www.nisc.com>* **2002**

- *IBZ International Bibliography of Periodical Literature* <http://www.saur.de> **2002**

- *Journal of Social Work Practice "Abstracts Section"* <http://www.carfax.co.uk/jsw-ad.htm> **2002**

- *Linguistics & Language Behavior Abstracts (LLBA)* <http://www.csa.com> **2002**

- *Natl Inst of Diabetes & Digestive & Kidney Diseases (NIDDK)* <http://www.niddk.nih.gov> **2002**

- *OT SEARCH <http://aotf.org>* **2002**

(continued)

- *Published International Literature On Traumatic Stress (The PILOTS Database) <http://www.ncptsd.org> (Abstracts Section)*. **2002**

- *Social Services Abstracts <http://www.csa.com>* **2002**

- *Social Work Abstracts <http://www.silverplatter.com/catalog/swab.htm>*. **2002**

- *Sociological Abstracts (SA) <http://www.csa.com>* **2002**

- *Worldwide Political Science Abstracts (formerly: Political Science & Government Abstracts) <http://www.csa.com>* **2002**

Special Bibliographic Notes related to special journal issues (separates) and indexing/abstracting:

- indexing/abstracting services in this list will also cover material in any "separate" that is co-published simultaneously with Haworth's special thematic journal issue or DocuSerial. Indexing/abstracting usually covers material at the article/chapter level.
- monographic co-editions are intended for either non-subscribers or libraries which intend to purchase a second copy for their circulating collections.
- monographic co-editions are reported to all jobbers/wholesalers/approval plans. The source journal is listed as the "series" to assist the prevention of duplicate purchasing in the same manner utilized for books-in-series.
- to facilitate user/access services all indexing/abstracting services are encouraged to utilize the co-indexing entry note indicated at the bottom of the first page of each article/chapter/contribution.
- this is intended to assist a library user of any reference tool (whether print, electronic, online, or CD-ROM) to locate the monographic version if the library has purchased this version but not a subscription to the source journal.
- individual articles/chapters in any Haworth publication are also available through the Haworth Document Delivery Service (HDDS).

International Perspectives on Disability Services: The Same But Different

CONTENTS

About the Contributors   xi

We Are Different and We Are the Same   1
    Francis K. O. Yuen

Disability Through the Lens of Culture   5
    Kristine D. Tower

Psychotherapy with Deaf and Hard of Hearing Individuals:
    Perceptions of the Consumer   23
    Carol B. Cohen

Life Participation Approaches to Aphasia:
    International Perspectives on Communication Rehabilitation   47
    Larry Boles
    Mimi Lewis

An Exploratory Study on Attitudes Toward Persons
    with Disabilities Among U.S. and Japanese
    Social Work Students   65
    Reiko Hayashi
    Mariko Kimura

Max versus *Max*: Disability-Related Services
    in the U.S. and Germany   87
    Ute C. Orgassa

Community Integration of Older People
    with Developmental Disabilities in Hong Kong   101
    Raymond Man-hung Ngan
    Mark Kin-yin Li
    Jacky Chau-kiu Cheung

Hmong Americans' Changing Views and Approaches
    Towards Disability: Shaman and Other Helpers   121
    Serge C. Lee
    Francis K. O. Yuen

Index   133

ABOUT THE EDITOR

Francis K. O. Yuen, DSW, ACSW, is Professor for the Division of Social Work at California State University in Sacramento. He is widely published in the areas of family health social work practice, disability, grant writing, program planning and evaluation, substance abuse, international social work, and services to refugees and immigrants. He is a member of several editorial boards, including those of the *Journal of Social Work in Disability & Rehabilitation* and the *Journal of Ethnic & Cultural Diversity in Social Work*. He has authored and edited many books, including several for The Haworth Press, Inc., such a *Family Health Social Work Practice: A Knowledge and Skills Casebook* (2003), *Family Health Social Work Practice with Children and Family* (In-Press), and the upcoming *Disability and Social Work Education: Practice and Policy Issues*. For over a decade, Dr. Yuen has been a consultant for local and government organizations on program evaluation, grant writing, proposal review, and human diversity issues.

About the Contributors

Larry Boles, PhD, CCC, is Associate Professor for the Department of Speech Pathology and Audiology at California State University, Sacramento. He has been a practicing speech-language pathologist for 20 years in California, Vermont, Arizona, and Hawaii. His clinical and research interests are in couple-based and conversation-based aphasia therapy, solution-focused aphasia therapy, confabulation and memory, conversation and discourse analysis, and transdisciplinary communication therapy. He has published and presented his research across the United States, in Hong Kong, Australia, and New Zealand.

Jacky Chau-kiu Cheung, PhD, in Sociology, is Senior Research Fellow at the City University of Hong Kong. His current research focuses on the quality of life of older and working people in a number of Chinese societies. Such a research direction builds on his past research on various life experiences in school, work, community, and institutional settings of young and older people. His research findings appear in a number of international social science journals.

Carol B. Cohen, PhD, LCSW-C, is Associate Professor for the Department of Social Work at Gallaudet University. Gallaudet University is the only liberal arts university in the world for deaf and hard of hearing students. Deafened as a young adult, Dr. Cohen's interests are in disability, deafness and clinical practice.

Reiko Hayashi, PhD, MSW, is Assistant Professor at University of Utah's College of Social Work. She is a member of the Commission on Disability and Persons with Disabilities under the Council on Social Work Education. Her research interests include environmental obstacles faced by people with disabilities, policies that facilitate the integration of people with disabilities into the community, and roles of social workers in the lives of people with disabilities.

Mariko Kimura, PhD, MSW, is Professor for the Department of Social Welfare, Faculty of Integrated Arts and Social Sciences at Japan Women's University. Her interests in community mental health and social work include innovative approach to psychosocial rehabilitation, partnership building among mental heath consumers and professionals, and cross-cultural comparative studies on Quality of Life of mental health consumers.

Serge C. Lee, PhD, MSW, is Associate Professor at California State University, Sacramento, Division of Social Work. His areas of specialization include multicultural social work practices, refugees and immigrants mental health issues, and research with diverse populations. He also has served as consultant to the Department of Health & Human Services, Substance Abuse and Mental Health Services Administration and the Office of Refugee Resettlement program.

Mimi Lewis, LCSW, DCSW, CSAC, is Lecturer for the Division of Social Work at California State University, Sacramento. Her interests in disability services include addiction social work in addition to her solution focused family work with Larry Boles. She has published her work in the *Asia-Pacific Journal of Speech, Language and Hearing*, and has presented her research across the United States, in Hong Kong, and Australia.

Kristine Tower, EdD, LCSW, is Assistant Professor of Social Work at the University of Nevada, Reno. Her background includes three decades as a consumer, activist, clinical social worker, and social work educator. Her primary area of practice is medical social work in rehabilitation, such as with survivors of spinal cord and brain injury. Her research interests are in disability culture, sexuality, technology, and special education. She is also a producer of several well-known documentary and television series on disability.

Mark Kin Yin Li, MSW, MPA, ACSW, is Lecturer for the Social Work Department at Hong Kong Baptist University. He has been a clinical supervisor for more than twenty years and is experienced in training, residential care, employment and empowerment of persons with intellectual deficiency. His other professional interests include gerontology, social security, social movement, and policy analysis. Li has published many articles and essays in the areas of social welfare, public policies, and politics of Hong Kong.

Raymond Man Hung Ngan, PhD, is Associate Professor (University Senior Lecturer) and former Associate Department Head at the Department of Applied Social Studies, City University of Hong Kong. He has been supervising social work students' field practicum in residential homes for persons with intellectual deficiency and family services. His other professional interests include employment and empowerment practices for socially handicapped groups, social security, social development, and gerontology. His writings have been published in refereed international journals and other journals in Chinese in Beijing, Taiwan and Hong Kong.

Ute C. Orgassa, PhD, Dipl Soz Paed, has studied social work in Germany and worked with persons with disabilities and their families in that capacity. She received her PhD at the University of Alabama and is currently living in Pasadena, CA. She is interested in disability issues in the context of the family experience.

Francis K. O. Yuen, DSW, ACSW, is Professor for the Division of Social Work at California State University, Sacramento. He has many books and journal publications in the areas of family health social work practice, disability, grant writing and program evaluation, substance abuse, international social work, and services to refugees and immigrants. He is a member of several editorial boards including the *Journal of Social Work in Disability & Rehabilitation* and the *Journal of Ethnic and Cultural Diversity in Social Work.*

We Are Different and We Are the Same

Francis K. O. Yuen

Chuang Tse (around 275 B.C.) a famous Chinese Philosopher, Naturalist, and one of the original Taoists, once told a story about nature and ability: A surprised one-legged bird said to a centipede, "I move with my one leg. It is so simple and easy. How could you move with that many legs?" The centipede responded, "Not a problem at all; it comes naturally. This is who I am and how I move." Just then a snake passed by and the centipede asked him, "I have many legs and you have none. How come you can move much faster than I can?" "Naturally. This is who I am and how I move. No legs are needed," the snake replied. "Look at the wind, it moves so fast and freely. It does not even have a body." The wind joined in and said, "Yes, I can move fast; but the eye can get to places yet faster. It reaches immediately to wherever the eye can see." The wind continued, "Our heart and mind are, in fact, much more amazing. They can reach any place that they wish to envision. As a wind, I could move trees and tumble houses. This is who I am and what I am capable of doing. Nature has its course and we all have our own unique niches and abilities. We are different and we are the same." Chung Tse may be an ancient figure who lived thousands of years ago. His insights, however, still have much to offer to our appreciation of our unique being and inherent capacities.

Francis K. O. Yuen is Professor, Division of Social Work, California State University-Sacramento, Sacramento, CA 95819-6090.

[Haworth co-indexing entry note]: "We Are Different and We Are the Same." Yuen, Francis K. O. Co-published simultaneously in *Journal of Social Work in Disability & Rehabilitation* (The Haworth Press, Inc.) Vol. 2, No. 2/3, 2003, pp. 1-3; and: *International Perspectives on Disability Services: The Same But Different* (ed: Francis K. O. Yuen) The Haworth Press, Inc., 2003, pp. 1-3. Single or multiple copies of this article are available for a fee from The Haworth Document Delivery Service [1-800-HAWORTH, 9:00 a.m. - 5:00 p.m. (EST). E-mail address: docdelivery@haworthpress.com].

http://www.haworthpress.com/store/product.asp?sku=J198
10.1300/J198v02n02_01

According to the United Nations (2002) over 500 million people or 10% of the world population are person with disabilities. Two thirds of them live in developing countries and many (80%) are poor. They live in isolated rural areas where services are both unavailable and inaccessible. In some developing countries, about 20% of the population are with some form of disability. The number of people with disabilities will continue to climb due to factors such as wars, disasters, increased birth rate, and poor medical care.

Disability does not discriminate. It is a reality for people of all races, genders, ages, social classes, and any other categories. Within these diverse contexts, there are also different perspectives on disability, as can be seen in the many disability-related social policies and services. These differences range from legal and human rights, designations, strategies, service activities, service availability and accessibility, to the philosophical stances toward disability. Many disciplines and professionals have engaged in researching and studying the various international aspects of disability and services to people with disability. As part of these on-going efforts, the following articles describe several disability related services in different cultural settings.

What is a disability culture? How could social work practitioners become sensitive or even competent in incorporating this culture into their practices? Kristine D. Tower discusses these important issues and suggests ways to infuse them into social work practice and education.

Carol B. Cohen conducts a qualitative study to explore the subjective experiences of deaf and hard-of-hearing individuals in psychotherapy. Her study examines culturally syntonic considerations for competent practice with this population. Effective communication, genuine acceptance, and empowerment orientation are among the important factors for the crucial experiential processes of treatment.

Participation Approach to Aphasia is a consumer-driven communication rehabilitation method that emphasizes re-engagement in life. Larry Boles and Mimi Lewis discuss their interdisciplinary application of this recently developed approach. It emphasizes the use of real-life interactions in the family and community to provide the context for the therapy.

Reiko Hayashi and Mariko Kimura compare the attitudes between Japanese and United States social work students' attitudes toward people with disability. The Modified Issues in Disabilities Scale was used to measure this attitude. Although both the Japanese and the U.S. students show positive attitudes, there are other subtle and important differences.

Using a fictional case example, Ute C. Orgassa contrasts the disability services in the United States and Germany. Following the case from birth to adulthood, the author identifies different social policies and services that may apply to a person with developmental disability. Subsequently, different life choices are available to the client.

Raymond Man-hung Ngan, Mark Kin-yin Li, and Jacky Chau-kiu Cheung study the community integration of 692 adults with developmental disabilities in Hong Kong. Although the older adults from the sample were knowledgeable about and were feeling accepted by their local communities, many had few interactions with the community. Greater support and facilitation are needed to promote greater community integration.

Serge C. Lee and Francis K. O. Yuen discuss how the concept of unique perceptions, beliefs, understanding, and respect of disability and persons with disabilities have evolved among Hmong Americans. Culturally and professionally competent practice with Hmong Americans requires the coordination, inclusion, and utilization of the family, shaman/shawoman, community leaders, Western medicine, and native folk beliefs.

REFERENCE

United Nations. (June 2002). The United Nations and Disabled Persons: The first 50 years. Available online: *http://www.un.org/esa/socdev/enable/dis50y01.htm*.

Disability Through the Lens of Culture

Kristine D. Tower

SUMMARY. Effective social work requires cultural sensitivity and competency. Until recently, there was little discussion of culture outside of the contexts of race or ethnicity. This article is an exploration of the key components of culture with application to the community of people with disabilities. The language, history, stigmatization, economic concerns, common behaviors, and practices of people with disabilities are highlighted. A literature review of sensitivity and competency in cross-cultural practice is provided. The article furnishes insights into the lived experience of disability. Suggestions to help practitioners reduce the risks of harm and improve service to this population are presented. Content on disability culture is proposed for social work educators to infuse into core curriculum or add to diversity electives. *[Article copies available for a fee from The Haworth Document Delivery Service: 1-800-HAWORTH. E-mail address: <docdelivery@haworthpress.com> Website: <http://www. HaworthPress.com> © 2003 by The Haworth Press, Inc. All rights reserved.]*

KEYWORDS. Disability, culture, sensitivity, strengths, technology, empowerment

---

Kristine D. Tower is Assistant Professor, University of Nevada, Reno, School of Social Work, Mail Stop 90, Reno, NV 89557-0068 (E-mail: drtower@nvbell.net).

[Haworth co-indexing entry note]: "Disability Through the Lens of Culture." Tower, Kristine D. Co-published simultaneously in *Journal of Social Work in Disability & Rehabilitation* (The Haworth Press, Inc.) Vol. 2, No. 2/3, 2003, pp. 5-22; and: *International Perspectives on Disability Services: The Same But Different* (ed: Francis K. O. Yuen) The Haworth Press, Inc., 2003, pp. 5-22. Single or multiple copies of this article are available for a fee from The Haworth Document Delivery Service [1-800-HAWORTH, 9:00 a.m. - 5:00 p.m. (EST). E-mail address: docdelivery@haworthpress.com].

INTRODUCTION

Teaching cultural sensitivity and competency is one of the most challenging aspects of social work education, yet no area of the curriculum is more important for the preparation of effective practitioners. Relationships between professionals and clients from different cultures are easily harmed by misunderstandings and unsupported assumptions (Lee & Greene, 1999). The Council on Social Work Education recognizes the impact of such barriers and appeals to educators to focus more intensively on multiculturalism and cultural competency (White, 1999).

One area that has only recently been discussed in social work is the cultural identity of people with disabilities. Shapiro asserted, "non-disabled Americans do not understand disabled ones" (1994, p. 3). It seems that social workers may not be an exception. Within the professional literature, it is unusual to find reference to a community of people with disabilities who comprise a true culture, and rarer still to find meaningful discourse on the nature of this important cultural identification (exceptions: Condeluci, 1995; Mackelprang & Salsgiver, 1999).

Impetus for the Article

After three decades as a consumer, activist, clinician (LCSW), and social work educator, I am adding my voice to the discussion of disability culture. I recognize, of course, that all of the first-hand experience, formal training, and practice wisdom of any individual could never be enough to fully represent this diverse culture. Furthermore, there are dangers involved when individuals attempt to define their own culture to others. I'm conscious that my personal experience as a woman with disabilities is not the norm. It is, however, worth the risk of inviting criticism about bias and overgeneralization if it promotes discussion about disability culture.

I have been teaching an intensive undergraduate social work course entitled "Disability: Social and Health Issues" for the past ten years (see syllabus in Gilson, 2002). Over 450 students (mostly non-disabled) have taken the course so far. In this class, I ask students to examine their feelings about disability openly and honestly. There are consistent themes in their comments before and after taking the class. In the beginning, most students admit to feeling "fear," "anxiety," or "dread" about disabilities and the people who have them. After completion, they report that they feel "comfortable" or "enthusiastic" about disability-related social work practice. Moreover, they have become less fearful about the possibility of disability in their own lives. I believe that their initiation into disability culture is the key to this transformation.

Regrettably, many social workers do not receive this type of orientation. A recent study of MSW-level practitioners revealed that less than 40% recalled content on disability in their social work training (Rittner, Nakanishi, Nackerud, & Hammons, 1999). It is time for educators to expand the way they view and teach about cultural diversity.

Culture Defined

Pinderhughes (1989) defined culture as "the sum total of ways of living developed by a group of human beings to meet biological and psychological needs" (p. 6). Values, norms, beliefs, behaviors, and traditions are among the key elements that function to sustain a culture within the larger society. Yet, some social work scholars continue to define culture solely within the context of ethnicity or race. Ethnic/racial groups are characterized by shared beliefs and practices, language, historical continuity, common origin, and physical attributes that differ from the majority (Alle-Corliss & Alle-Corliss, 1999). Notice the similarities to the characteristics of disability culture. The origins for all disabilities are few: accidents, illnesses, or genetics. People with disabilities often have physical attributes that differ from the majority. They share a common history and mutual language. Further, they have similar economic concerns, collective feelings of stigmatization, and typical norms of behavior. This article examines disability through the lens of culture with attention to the unifying elements that draw individuals with disabilities together as a community.

Cultural Sensitivity and Competence

Some scholars propose that social workers should approach all diverse clients with universal *cultural sensitivity*, such as finding common ground, respecting individuality, and having a willingness to learn (Hatfield & Lefley, 1993). Others believe that *cultural competence*, like possessing knowledge, skills, and values for working within a given population, is the best cross-cultural practice (Weaver, 1999). Both methods are useful at certain times when working with people with disabilities. In some cases, practitioners should avoid posturing as experts. In other situations, social workers need a high level of specific knowledge in order to be helpful.

Helping professionals must at least be knowledgeable enough to do no harm. When practitioners approach clients with misperceptions and stereotypes about disability, they may be the source of pain to the very people they want to help (Condelucci, 1995; Shapiro, 1994). Improved sensitivity and competency relieves some of the concerns that social workers may have about inadvertently hurting their clients. Learning about disability culture increases confidence about service to this community and results in strengths-based practices (Saleebey, 1996; Russo, 1999).

Strengths-Based

Studies indicate that many social workers are not sufficiently skilled to be effective helpers for people with disabilities and their families (Petr & Barney, 1993). Without proper training, social workers tend to view disability in excessively negative terms, primarily as physical and/or mental defects. It may come as a surprise, but living with disability is rarely as tragic as people expect. Vash wrote, "Ultimately, we do more than transcend our pain and suffering. We don't repudiate it and leave it behind; we bring it with us, transformed from an awful catastrophe into a valued treasure of experience" (1995, p. 36). Too often, social workers lack understanding about surviving and thriving through adversity (McMillen, 1999). They fail to recognize disability as a form of human variability that for many people is a source of pride, personal growth, identification, and affiliation. The Deaf community, for example, asserts that deafness is an alternative culture and lifestyle, not a physical limitation (Luey, Glass, & Elliott, 1995).

DISABILITY AS CULTURE

There is an ongoing philosophical debate by disability rights leaders about the value of identifying people with disabilities as a social minority group (Mackelprang & Salsgiver, 1999). In particular, the arguments against identification are that such assignments perpetuate a "victim status" and further promote the stigmatization of disability (Phillips, 1985, p. 48). On the other hand, there are known benefits of group affiliation (i.e., advocacy, strength in numbers) and cultural identification (i.e., peer support, pride) that emerges from relationships between people with disabilities (Shapiro, 1994). Despite the arguments against minority identification, there is little debate that disability culture exists.

Lathrop (1999, p. 25) said, "I'm afraid my view of disability culture is similar to Supreme Court Justice Paul Steven's famous definition of obscenity: 'I can't define it, but I know it when I see it.'" Actually, it is easier to find evidence of a tangible disability culture than he suggests. During the past two decades there has been a proliferation of disability-related activities: political gatherings, sports/recreation events, conferences, arts, entertainment, support, and socialization groups (including dating services), magazines, newsletters, Internet web-sites and chat rooms. On-line self-help groups are emerging (Finn, 1999). There is actually an Institute on Disability Culture (www.dimenet.com/disculture). Through such channels, the disability community is spreading and becoming global.

Wade (1992) presented a keynote address about disability culture to the Corporation on Disabilities and Telecommunications, which included this excerpt:

> Disability culture. *Say what?* Aren't disabled people just isolated victims of nature or circumstance? Yes and no. True, we are far too often isolated. Locked away in the pits, closets, and institutions of enlightened societies everywhere. But there is a growing consciousness among us: *that* is not acceptable. Because there is always an underground. Notes get passed along among the survivors. And the notes we're passing these days say, "there's power in difference. Power. Pass the word." (p. 37)

People from within the culture are redefining the terms of living with disability and the new definition includes power. It also includes pride. The sense of pride is illustrated in the culture's celebration of the community's heroes and ancestors. Until recently, people with disabilities were considered "invisibles" and their history denied (Wade, 1992, p. 37). New disability culture demands a re-examination of history, so leaders with disabilities are acknowledged for their contributions. To illustrate, when a bronze statue of President Franklin Roosevelt was unveiled, advocates protested emphatically about his carefully disguised wheelchair. They rejected the notion that polio was shameful or that it detracted from FDR's remarkable presidency. Disability history is enriched by the life of this president and to minimize his experience with polio is disrespectful to people within the culture.

Who Comprises Disability Culture?

It is generally accepted that nearly one in every five Americans (19.4%) has a disability (Kraus, Stoddard, & Gilmartin, 1996). Regardless of the measurement used, people with disabilities constitute the largest specific population group in the United States. Estimates vary widely on the total number of Americans with disabilities but all could be considered *members* of the culture, regardless of whether or not individuals choose to align themselves with it. People don't have to be active participants to reap the benefits, or conversely, to suffer the consequences of being identified with a cultural group.

The National Center for the Dissemination of Disability Research (1998) reported that there were 54 million people with some level of disability in the U.S. But, the culture encompasses more people than just those with disabilities. Family members, particularly parents and spouses, comprise some of the most influential and active sub-groups within the larger disability community. In addition, there are many human service professionals who have a strong cultural identification with this population.

Unity and Difference

There are innumerable disability-related groups that bring people with similar experiences and needs together. They range from local independent support groups to international networks. Cumulatively, disability groups form the largest social and political constituency in the U.S. (Shapiro, 1994). Their strength has been most evident when they joined together as a combined force, like when they rallied for the Americans With Disabilities Act. Speaking in unison, they have the power to break down social barriers. Unfortunately, divisiveness between the groups occasionally impedes the success of the disability rights movement. Among the major disability sub-groups are: (1) consumer organizations representing people with disabilities in general; (2) research and policy groups; (3) groups for specific types of disabilities; (4) groups for specific age cohorts; (5) wheelchair athletes; (6) veterans with disabilities; and (7) families of people with disabilities. It is important for social workers to understand the cultural dynamics between these groups. While they may be unified when it truly matters, they don't always agree about tactics or values. For example, consumer groups of people with mental disorders may have very different goals than support groups for their family members. The former usually embraces independence as their highest priority. Families are generally more concerned about safety. The goals make sense from each perspective, but it is easy to see how they may clash.

One advocacy group called ADAPT sometimes uses non-violent civil disobedience (sit-ins, demonstrations) to increase public awareness about injustice toward people with disabilities. Some groups find these approaches too radical. Other conflicts exist about fundraising tactics like the Jerry Lewis telethon. The telethon or poster child approach to raising money is a quarrelsome topic. Proponents defend it as a successful way to raise money for research, client services, or public education (Fields, 1999). Opponents insist that no amount of money justifies perpetuating the image of people with disabilities as pitiful or doomed (Wang, 1993).

Another divisive issue within the community is the topic of physician-assisted suicide. Many individuals favor end-of-life choices, but several groups have come out in opposition to support for euthanasia. An advocacy group, NOT DEAD YET, asserts that too many people with non-terminal disabilities, like spinal cord injuries, are given the option of dying instead of the proper services and supports to make life worth living (Johnson, 1999b; Toy, 1999).

There is a long-standing conflict about the issue of communication methods among people who are deaf or hard-of-hearing. The Deaf community is generally opposed to learning oral language and asserts that sign language is the primary unifying element of the culture (Luey, Glass, & Elliott, 1995). People who are hard-of-hearing usually don't learn sign language and prefer alternative methods to enhance communication (including lip reading, augmentive devices, or surgical procedures). This may seem like a simple matter of personal choice, but among many in Deaf culture, the issue of oral language is divisive. People who talk, "talkies," are rarely accepted within the inner circle of leadership within the Deaf community. This tension is further demonstrated in the debates about cochlear implants (a surgical procedure) to correct hearing deficits. Deaf people are strongly opposed to the implants because they represent the loss of culture.

Disability groups may differ philosophically, but they are united in their support of crucial political issues. There is consensus about the need for increased resources for independent living and home-based care versus institutionalization. Many are lobbying for consumer autonomy and increased resources for personal care services, access to communication, respite, transportation, employment, accessible housing, and comprehensive health care.

Clearly, it is not necessary to find perpetual agreement among people with disabilities to identify them as a distinctive cultural group. Although each group has its own culture, there is a collective culture as well. It is based, in part, by their long common history as "second-class citizens" (Eisenberg, Griggins, & Duval, 1982, p. 1).

A COMMON HISTORY

Living conditions are improving, but it is a mistake for social workers to overlook the bleak and contentious history that has been the cornerstone of disability culture. Most adults with developmental disabilities can recall accepted practices in schools or institutions that would be considered cruel and inhumane by current standards (e.g., slapping, pinching, isolation, and lengthy restraint). History is replete with horror stories of people enduring imprisonment, forced sterilization, involuntary lobotomies, and other atrocities, such as bloodletting and purging (Winzer, 1993). It hasn't been that long since the end of one the darkest periods in history for people with disabilities, the Eugenics era. Beginning near the turn of the 20th century and lasting until the mid-1950s, a number of influential scientists, including Alexander Graham Bell and Henry Goddard, asserted that the human gene pool was tainted by individuals with low intellect and/or immoral character. During their 50 years of prominence, the eugenicists forced over 30,000 people into involuntary sterilization in the U.S. alone. Adolph Hitler embraced the rationale of the Eugenics movement and used it to justify outright genocide.

Until the early 1970s, educational scholars were convinced that large numbers of students were uneducable and should be denied access to public education. Neither children nor their parents had due process rights. As recently as the late 1980s, social work literature blamed innocent parents for causing certain types of developmental disabilities (Turner, 1986). The double-bind theory of schizophrenia, for instance, asserted that mothers caused their children to become mentally ill by sending them mixed messages. Bruno Bettleheim called parents of children with autism "refrigerator parents" because they were believed to be so emotionally cold toward their children that they caused this devastating mental disorder (Turnbull & Turnbull, 1996). Since parents were considered culpable, they were discredited and discouraged from participating in the children's treatment. It wasn't until the advent of new medical technology, like MRI and PET scans, that the structural changes in the brain, caused by genetics, viruses, or other pathogens, became evident. Modern science now recognizes that the brain, like any other organ of the body, is subject to illness and injury. Finally, the myths about parental causation are starting to fade. Social workers must be aware, however, that the emotional scars caused by enduring such blame run deep. Moreover, parents often feel guilty about their children's disabilities whether there is just cause or not. Practitioners need to be sensitive to these feelings.

Two Steps Forward

The most significant historical event in the evolution of disability culture has been the independent living movement. One of the earliest disability rights legislation was passed into law in 1975, known as the Education of All Handicapped Children's Act (EHA). This legislation ensured the rights of all children to a free and appropriate public education in the least restrictive environment. It has evolved since then to promote greater inclusion of all children into regular (*integrated*), *as opposed to special (segregated)* education. Renamed IDEA, the act also provides early intervention services for young children with developmental disabilities. In 1990, the Americans With Disabilities Act (ADA) became law. It was enacted to promote equal access to jobs and public accommodations. While the policies are signs of continued progress, they are tenuous victories. Despite these advancements, there are ongoing, acrimonious debates about the rights of people with disabilities to live with the same level of freedom as others (NASW News, 1999). Conservative legislators protest the costs associated with federal education laws, while concurrently fighting against unfunded mandates, like the ADA. Many view these policies as compassionate excess. So far, courts and legislators have consistently voted against people with disabilities in the vast majority (86% to 92%) of individual civil rights cases testing the new federal laws (Porter, 1998). The past is subject to repetition unless concerned people, including social workers, take action to guard against the erosion of these basic human rights.

A MUTUAL LANGUAGE

A sustaining element of disability culture is its language. People with disabilities share a common vocabulary consisting of an alphabet-soup of programs and policy acronyms, medical jargon, and friendly "in-group" slang. As with other diverse cultures, involvement in this community requires basic understanding of the accepted nomenclature. Suggestions are provided which should be useful for social workers in a variety of contexts. Use caution, however, because some individuals, both with and without disabilities, may still be offended by these terms. It is also necessary to point out that language, like other aspects of culture, "is in reality fluid, constantly evolving" (Kenyatta & Tai, 1997, p. 176). Some terms are still in common usage among the public, but are rejected by the disability community (e.g., *handicapped*). Other terms have generated debate, but there is no agreement (e.g., *able-bodied, mentally retarded*). In fact, the whole issue of political correctness is being challenged.

Social workers should err on the side of empowerment language (Rappaport, 1985). The term *disability* continues to dominate in the community's literature and use of "people-first" language has been widely promoted and institutionalized (Mackelprang & Salsgiver, 1999). It is correct to say *people, persons, or children with disabilities, a woman with cerebral palsy, a child with intellectual impairment,* for example. In each case, human beings precede their descriptions. Conversely, *disabled man* and *a FAS child* are not examples of empowerment language. This distinction between using *disability* as an adjective or as part of a prepositional phrase is important. People with disabilities are *people* first. It is also not proper to speak in general terms such as, *the disabled* or *the mentally ill*. Such language has *us-versus-them* or *those people* overtones.

There is an exception to the emphasis on people-first language that comes from the Deaf community. They embrace *D*eaf culture with a capital *D*! There is no movement to change the terminology. It is acceptable to say *Deaf person* or *Deaf child*. The term "deaf" conveys an absence of hearing, whereas "Deaf" implies community membership (Luey, Glass, & Elliott, 1995). This variation is an example of the uniqueness of each group within the larger disability community (Shapiro, 1994).

In popular publications, like *The Ragged Edge, Mouth, and New Mobility*, the language is often candid and provocative. Some authors refer to themselves as *gimps or crips*. They use these monikers in two ways; (1) as "in-group" slang, or (2) in protest to stereotypes about disability. It is a healthy rebellion, like gay men and lesbian women use when they celebrate the term *queer* (e.g., Queer Nation). It is also an expression of pride and group affiliation. Such terms, however, are generally inappropriate for social workers (without disabilities).

Outdated terms, such as *crippled, incurable, invalid, mongoloid, and mute,* have fallen into disuse because they're ugly overstatements. Although the term *physically challenged* is believed to be a politically correct alternative, it is not used by people with disabilities in any of the community's literature. Personally, it seems like an attempt to gloss over the reality of life with disability, a sign of discomfort. From the standpoint of consumers, practitioners who are too uncomfortable to say the word *disability,* are incapable of being at ease with people who have them. This holds true for other avoidance phrases, such as *inconvenienced, handi-capable, alternatively-able, or able-disabled.* People don't use such language to describe themselves nor should social workers.

Handicapped, as mentioned, is another problem word. In 16th century England and colonial America, poor laws established the criteria for those individuals who were considered worthy of assistance, including people who were unable to work due to a disabling condition (Rothman, 2003). Only they were allowed to sit with *cap-in-hand* to beg. Other negative connotations are associated with this term. Handicaps are used in gambling circles to equalize otherwise losing bets. People with disabilities reject the notion that they are losers.

The term *special needs* is frequently used to describe children with disabilities, but it isn't an appropriate term to use when discussing adults. It is too paternalistic to be accepted among adults and probably shouldn't be used for children either. The term is contrary to the values the community is trying to convey. They reject the notion that they are special. People with disabilities want to be treated like ordinary people, not elevated or reduced in status in comparison to others. Table 1 contains additional guidelines to aid social workers.

COMMON ECONOMIC CONCERNS

Currently and historically, people with disabilities are among the poorest and least educated Americans (Kopels, 1995). The combination of inadequate training and discrimination in hiring practices is reflected in a staggering unemployment rate from 68% to 88%. In a Harris Poll conducted in 1994, it was reported that 69% of people with disabilities aged 16 to 64 were not working. Of those that were, only 20% worked full time. When working, people earn 35% less than their non-disabled co-workers, a very troubling statistic given that it holds consistently through all levels of education (in Medgyesi, 1996).

The primary reason for the passage of the ADA was recognition that these citizens comprise the most economically disadvantaged group in the United States. "Across the board, the poverty rate increases substantially when a householder has a disability" (Kaye, LaPlante, & Wenger, 1996, p. 3). The rates of poverty and unemployment are higher among women with disabilities than their male counterparts. People with the

TABLE 1. Empowerment Language

GOOD	AVOID
person with a disability, consumer, survivor (use cautiously; acceptable in some groups, such as cancer survivors).	*disabled* person, handicapped, crippled, physically challenged, special, *the* disabled
has . . . (e.g., has M.S.; has epilepsy)	victim, or victim of . . . afflicted with . . . stricken with . . . suffers from . . .
uses a wheelchair in a wheelchair	wheelchair-bound confined to a wheelchair prisoner of . . .
segregated school separate bus, school paratransit system	special school special van
inclusion (involves proper supports for students with disabilities to participate in regular education)	mainstreaming (involved integrating students with disabilities without proper supports; was not very effective)
living with . . . (e.g., HIV/AIDS)	dying from . . .
intellectually impaired intellectual disorder	mentally retarded
deaf; hearing impaired (Do not use these terms interchangeably.)	deaf-mute
accessible parking wheelchair access	handicapped parking disabled ramps, seating
	in spite of his disability overcame her handicaps . . . is the least disabled person I ever knew

most severe disabilities have the highest rates of unemployment and poverty overall (Kopels, 1995).

It was hoped that the ADA would result in greater numbers of people with disabilities entering the workforce. Certainly, this important civil rights legislation has improved environmental conditions, particularly in the area of public accommodations, such as widening doors and providing ramps for wheelchair access. However, in the four years after the law took effect, the unemployment rate of all people with disabilities actually increased by an average of 4% (U.S. Census, 1996). It appears that misconceptions and prejudice are not as easily eliminated as architectural barriers. Economic injustice will persist as long as employers continue to devalue the contribution of people with disabilities.

STIGMATIZATION

Although pride within the culture is increasing as stereotypes diminish, there is no point in denying that stigma persists. The term *stigma* refers to an attribute that is unusual and that is deeply disparaging. "By definition, we believe the person with a stigma is not quite human. On this assumption we exercise varieties of discrimination through which we effectively, if often unthinkingly, reduce his life chances" (Goffman, 1963, p. 5). The more defensively people with disabilities react to their situations, the more assured others are that illness or injury is just retribution for some wrongdoing.

No one is immune from stigmatization. Film star Kathleen Turner (*Romancing the Stone*) recently announced that she has rheumatoid arthritis. At times, she takes steroid medications that cause her to look bloated. She kept her condition private until the Hollywood gossip mill began speculating that she had a drinking problem. When she came out publicly, her job offers dried up. She was shocked to find, "I was better off with people thinking I had a drinking problem than to think I was ill. I could get hired with a drinking problem. They wouldn't hire me if they thought I was disabled" (*The View*, 11/20/97). Ms. Turner was stunned by the stigmatization of having rheumatoid arthritis. It is a harsh reality that people with disabilities have always known.

NORMS OF BEHAVIOR: RESPONDING TO LIFE WITH DISABILITY

Until recently, the limited options for surviving with disability required that individuals conform their behaviors to fit within societal expectations. Those options are expanding now and the norms of conduct within the disability community are changing too. Until recently there were only two potential ways for people with disabilities to respond to their life conditions: acquiescence or normalization (Phillips, 1985). *Acquiescence* means resigning to stereotypes about disability, allowing others to view people with disabilities as helpless, dependent, or objects of sympathy and pity. Disability activists point repugnantly to the telethon approach of fundraising and public education as an example. This strategy demands the sacrifice of dignity in order to gain social acceptance. *Normalization* is the flip side of acquiescence. It is another strategy that has been challenged lately. Normalization consists of denying one's disability and trying to attain the appearance of normality regardless of the personal cost. People are encouraged to "try harder" to overcome their disabilities and to adopt the expectations of non-disabled people (Phillips, 1985, p. 45). This includes avoiding wheelchairs in favor of walking, despite how slow or painful that effort might be. Government programs like Vocational Rehabilitation and Social Security strongly support this perspective, as evidenced by their measures of success, full-time employment. The fallacy behind normalization is that this type of success is rarely possible to sustain and true acceptance is seldom attained.

Some people continue to use acquiescence or normalization as their strategies for living with disability. Although they're polar opposites, these responses have something in common. Both are embedded in the belief that there are no other options. Acquiescence works because modern society usually accepts some responsibility for caring for its most vulnerable members. But this strategy lasts only as long as the person is willing to behave according to expectations; namely, to be good and to have a non-complaining attitude. Normalization requires a total commitment to overcoming disability as opposed to living with disability. This strategy comes with an expensive price tag. When all of one's energy is spent keeping up the appearance of normality, there is little left for enjoying life. A strenuous 40-hour work schedule with no flexibility or accommodations, for example, may deplete the energy required to maintain a healthy family life.

With the rise of the disability rights movement, other strategies have emerged that have expanded the definition of personal and social success: adaptation, re-negotiation, and inversion (Phillips, 1985). *Adaptation* involves modifying the environment, removing barriers, and accommodating needs. This strategy includes utilization of assistive technology (e.g., voice-activated or eye-gaze computers, environmental controls), and other supports, including personal care attendants. The passage of the ADA was a definite step in meeting the goals of this strategy. *Re-negotiation* involves changing the social definitions of success and normality. For example, the maximization of one's potential regardless of societal expectations is one goal. Under this strategy, success may be defined by the ability to participate in volunteer work, attend college, write poetry, be politically active, or simply survive. *Inversion* involves the rejection of stereotypes about disability (Phillips, 1985). The goal of this strategy is to change attitudes and thereby eliminate social obstacles. This conduct involves celebrating individuality and diversity, forcing society to view people with disabilities as people to respect or detest, but not pity or devalue. Outspoken use of terms like *gimp* is an example.

Like other marginalized groups in American society today, people with disabilities are demanding more respect, dignity, and freedom.

Their actions are healthy alternatives to the previous strategies that often led to passivity or failure. When working with individuals with disabilities, it is important to be aware of their strategies of adaptation. Typically, a person will not rely on just one approach but will utilize a combination of strategies depending on the situation, context, or stage of rehabilitation. Progressive social workers will promote those strategies that foster the highest quality of life for their clients.

THE FUTURE OF DISABILITY CULTURE: IMPLICATIONS FOR SOCIAL WORKERS

Alinsky (1971) asserted that it is revolution, not evolution, that brings about social change. The changes in opportunities and living conditions for people with disabilities have been nothing short of revolutionary. There is concern, however, among the leaders of the disability community that the political momentum built during the 1970s through the 1990s will be lost on a new generation of people with disabilities that won't remember the extraordinary hardships of the pre-movement days. The fight for equality and justice hasn't ended. Activists are still engaged in Supreme Court battles, including the Olmstead case, in which advocates are fighting to keep states from forcing people into institutions in order to receive medical support services (Johnson, 1999a). The hard work that went into developing policies to ensure the least restrictive environment is being undermined. It is a sad irony but conflicts like this continue to strengthen disability culture because each assault reaffirms the commitment of group members.

In contrast, there are other new trends in disability culture that bode well for the future. The literature is filled with discussion about interpersonal relationships, intimacy, parenting, information and communication technology, sports, and recreation. The next generation of young people with disabilities is entering a world that is open to any possibilities. Reasonable accommodations and assistive technology have proven to be the great equalizers in education, employment, transportation, and social life. For long-time veterans of disability culture, new developments offer a rediscovery of lost abilities, like working or enjoying intimacy. The renowned physicist, Stephen Hawking, who has advanced stage ALS (Lou Gehrig's disease), described the new technology as a lifeline for expressing his "human-ness" (Alliance for Technology Access, 1994, viii). It allows him to remain active within the scientific community and maintain the personal relationships that give meaning to his life.

Progressive social workers understand the significance of disability culture as a tool for empowerment. As people come together to share their strengths and problems, relationships are built, new resources are discovered, and the power of individuals and the group increases. Eventually, larger systems (i.e., bureaucratic, political) are influenced to change. True social progress, like the ADA and IDEA, results from this grass-roots approach.

To become part of the process, social workers must be willing to learn about the issues that drive the community, such as the history of oppression, stigmatization, and poverty. They need to understand the human response to those offenses, including the coping behavior of individuals and the dynamics of disability groups. Knowledge of the language and communication models, emerging technology, and political issues are also helpful. While this article touches on all of those issues, social workers may deepen their understanding by getting involved with local consumer organizations (e.g., Centers for Independent Living, Alliance for Mentally Ill). Subscriptions to popular publications will provide information on the national and international levels. Recent social work journals and texts are important reading (see Mackelprang & Salsgiver, 1999). For a general resource guide, Spinal Network (Corbet, 2000) is an essential tool.

For practitioners and educators who already identify with disability culture, the need for increasing theoretical discussion is evident. Continued studies on the effects of disability-group affiliation, peer counseling, cultural identification, and on-line support services are needed. A broad study of the disability training and knowledge of practicing social workers is in order. Finally, research is needed on social work educators' readiness to teach students about disability and the related culture. It is tragic that many social workers graduate without the cultural sensitivity and competency needed to serve this community. As informed case managers, advocates, group facilitators, clinicians, agency supervisors, administrators, educators, and private citizens, social workers have important contributions to make to the future of this vital culture.

REFERENCES

Alinsky, S. (1971). *Rules for radicals: A pragmatic primer for realistic radicals.* New York, Random House.

Alle-Corliss, L., & Alle-Corliss, R. (1999). *Advanced practice in human service agencies: Issues, trends, and treatment perspectives.* Belmont, CA: Brooks/Cole Publishing.

Alliance for Technology Access (1994). *Computer resources for people with disabilities: A guide to exploring today's assistive technology.* Alameda: CA. Hunter House Publishing.

Condeluci, A. (1995). *Interdependence: The route to community.* (2nd ed.). Winter Park, FL: G.R. Press.

Corbet, B. (2000). *Spinal Network: The total wheelchair resource book.* (3rd ed.). Malibu, CA: New Mobility Publications.

Eisenberg, M., Griggins, C., & Duval, R. (1982). *Disabled people as second-class citizens.* New York: Springer Publishing.

Fields, C. (1999). The 1.5 billion dollar man. *WE: The Lifestyle Magazine for People with Disabilities, Their Families and Friends, 3*(2), 22-27.

Finn, J. (1999). An exploration of helping processes in an online self-help group focusing on issues of disability. *Health and Social Work, 24*(3), 220-231.

Gilson, S. F. (2002). *Integrating disability content in social work education: A curriculum resource.* Alexandria, VA: Council on Social Work Education, 130-142.

Goffman, E. (1963). *Stigma.* Englewood Cliffs, N J: Prentice Hall Publishing.

Hatfield, A. B., & Lefley, H. P. (1993). *Surviving mental illness: Stress, coping, and adaptation.* New York: Guilford Press.

Johnson, M. (1999a). Our supremely defining moment. *Ragged Edge, May/June,* 9.

Johnson, M. (1999b). Quadriplegic dies after respirator removed: Activist group denied restraining order. *Ragged Edge, September/October,* 11.

Kaye, H. S., LaPlante, M., & Wenger, B. L. (1996). Trends in disability rates in the United States, 1970-1994. *Disability Statistics Abstracts, 17,* 1-6.

Kenyatta, M., & Tai, R. H. (Eds.). (1997). Ethnicity and education forum: What difference does difference make? *Harvard Educational Review, 67*(2), 169-187.

Kopels, S. (1995). The Americans With Disabilities Act: A tool to combat poverty. *Journal of Social Work Education, 31*(3), 337-346.

Kraus, L., Stoddard, S., & Gilmartin, D. (1996). *Chartbook on disability in the United States.* Washington, DC: National Institute on Disability and Rehabilitation Research.

Lathrop, D. (1999). Finding the art and soul of disability. *New Mobility, 10(70),* 24-27.

Lee, M & Greene, G (1999). A social constructivist framework for integrating cross-cultural issues in teaching clinical social work. *Journal of Social Work Education, 35*(1), 21-38.

Luey, H. S., Glass, L., & Elliott, H. (1995). Hard-of-hearing or Deaf: Issues of ears, language, culture, and identity. *Social Work, 40*(2), 177-181.

Mackelprang, R., & Salsgiver, R. (1999). *Disability: A diversity model approach in human service practice.* Belmont, CA: Brooks/Cole Publishing.

McMillen, J. (1999). Better for it: How people benefit from adversity. *Social Work, 44,* 455-468.

Medgyesi, V. (1996). The chrome ceiling. *New Mobility, 37,* 26-30.

NASW News. (Sept. 1999). Court backs option for mentally disabled. *NASW News, 44*(6), p. 6.

National Center for the Dissemination of Disability Research (1998). How many Americans have disabilities? *The Research Exchange, 3,* 3.

Petr, C., & Barney, D. (1993). Reasonable efforts for children with disabilities: The parents' perspective. *Social Work, 38,* 247-254.

Phillips, M. (1985). Try harder: The experience of disability and the dilemma of normalization. *The Social Science Journal, 22,* 47-57.

Pinderhughes, E. (1989*). Understanding race, ethnicity, and power: The key to efficacy in clinical practice.* New York: Free Press.

Porter, R. (1998). Employees lose most ADA suits, study shows. *Trial, 34*(9), 16-19.

Public Law 94-142 (1977). Education for All Handicapped Children Act of 1975. Federal Register (August 23, 1977).

Rappaport, J. (1985). The power of empowerment language. *Social Policy, 17*, 15-21.

Rittner, B., Nakanishi, M., Nackerud, L., & Hammons, K. (1999). How MSW graduates apply what they learned about diversity to their work with small groups. *Journal of Social Work Education, 35*(3), 421-431.

Rothman, J. C. (2003). Social work practice across disability. Boston, MA: Allyn & Bacon Publishing.

Russo, R. J. (1999). Applying a strengths-based practice approach in working with people with developmental disabilities and their families. *Families in Society, 80*(1), 25-33.

Saleebey, D. (1996). The strengths perspective in social work practice: Extensions and cautions. *Social Work, 41*(3), 296-305.

Shapiro, J. P. (1994). *No pity: People with disabilities forging a new civil rights movement.* New York: Random House Publishing.

The View (11/20/97). Interview with Kathleen Turner and Barbara Walters, ABC Television.

Toy, A. (1999). Assisted suicide: Issues of death and life. *New Mobility, 10*(72), 34-42.

Turnbull, H. R., & Turnbull, A. P. (1996). *Families, professionals, and exceptionality: A special partnership.* (2nd ed.). New York: Merrill Publishing.

Turner, F. (1986). *Social work treatment: Interlocking theoretical approaches.* (2nd ed.). New York: The Free Press.

U.S. Census Bureau. (1996). *Disability labor force status of persons 16 to 64.* Washington, DC: U.S. Government Printing Office.

Vash, C. L. (1995). From transcendence to transformation. *New Mobility, 6*(22), 36-37.

Wade, C. (1992). Disability culture rap. *The Disability Rag, September/October*, p. 37.

Wang, C. (1993). Culture, meaning and disability: Injury prevention campaigns and the production of stigma. In M. Nagler (Ed.), *Perspectives on disability.* (2nd ed.). Palo Alto, CA: Health Markets Research.

Weaver, H. (1999). Indigenous people and the social work profession: Defining culturally competent services. *Social Work, 44*(3), 217-225.

White, B. (1999). Quality in social work education. *CSWE Reporter, 47*, 1.

Winzer, M. A. (1993). *The history of special education: From isolation to integration.* Washington, DC: Gallaudet University Press.

Psychotherapy with Deaf and Hard of Hearing Individuals: Perceptions of the Consumer

Carol B. Cohen

SUMMARY. This qualitative study explored the subjective experiences of deaf and hard-of-hearing individuals in psychotherapy. Which culturally syntonic considerations are necessary for effective psychotherapy with deaf and hard-of-hearing individuals? The findings support the literature on multiculturalism and deafness that entail effective communication, empowerment processes, cultural sensitivity, therapist role flexibility, the imparting of information, and the development of a positive therapeutic relationship. The data focuses on the experience of communicating rather than focusing solely on the acquisition of content as well as the understanding the clinical dynamics of the transcultural relationship in order to make effective use of the social work relationship in treatment. The findings of this study add richness and depth to the existing literature on psychotherapy, with emphasis on the experiential processes of treatment. *[Article copies available for a fee from The Haworth Document Delivery Service: 1-800-HAWORTH. E-mail address: <docdelivery@ haworthpress.com> Website: <http://www.HaworthPress.com> © 2003 by The Haworth Press, Inc. All rights reserved.]*

Carol B. Cohen is affiliated with the Department of Social Work, Gallaudet University, 800 Florida Avenue, NE, Washington, DC 20002.

[Haworth co-indexing entry note]: "Psychotherapy with Deaf and Hard of Hearing Individuals: Perceptions of the Consumer." Cohen, Carol B. Co-published simultaneously in *Journal of Social Work in Disability & Rehabilitation* (The Haworth Press, Inc.) Vol. 2, No. 2/3, 2003, pp. 23-46; and: *International Perspectives on Disability Services: The Same But Different* (ed: Francis K. O. Yuen) The Haworth Press, Inc., 2003, pp. 23-46. Single or multiple copies of this article are available for a fee from The Haworth Document Delivery Service [1-800-HAWORTH, 9:00 a.m. - 5:00 p.m. (EST). E-mail address: docdelivery@haworthpress.com].

10.1300/J198v02n02_03

KEYWORDS. Deafness, multiculturalism, qualitative research, communication, transcultural processes, empowerment

This qualitative study explored the subjective experiences of deaf and hard-of-hearing individuals in psychotherapy. Two questions guided the study: Which considerations are necessary for effective psychotherapy with deaf and hard of hearing individuals and are there specific techniques or processes that are culturally syntonic in psychotherapy with deaf and hard-of-hearing individuals?

RATIONALE

Many researchers contend that deaf and hard-of-hearing individuals can be viewed as members of both a cultural group and a marginalized population (Glickman, 1996a; Lane, Hoffmeister, & Bahan, 1996; Corker, 1994). Due in large part to their different mode of communication–visual/spatial, rather than oral–this takes into account isolation, discrimination, and unequal access to resources, opportunities, and services in the dominant society. There have been numerous accounts in this population of misdiagnosis and inaccessibility to adequate mental health services (Dubow, Geer, & Strauss, 1992; Falicov, 1995; 1999; Steinberg, Sullivan, & Loew, 1998; Steinberg, Sullivan, & Lowe, 1999; Sussman & Brauer, 1999). The dynamics of mistreatment are complex: lack of appropriate communication between the client and service provider, providers' prejudices and biases; and their lack of cultural understanding of deafness. This lack of accessibility, cultural insensitivity, and inappropriate mental health services have been compounded by the paucity of training facilities that educate clinicians, therapists, social workers, and psychologists on the special issues and needs of deaf clients (Vernon, 1995). The intent of this research was to break from hearing models of values in order to understand the stories of deaf and hard-of-hearing consumers of psychotherapy. This research is one of the few inductive studies that focus on a consumer perspective.

MEANING OF DEAFNESS

In the discourse on disability, there are several different constructions for viewing disability, and in particular, deafness. The medical model views disability from the perspective of functional limitations and thus views the deaf individual as deficient in the ability to hear and possibly the ability to speak. The economic model views disability in relation to the individual's ability to work and function in society. Perhaps the most devastating consequences of having a disability are the stereotypes and prejudices associated with disability (Brzuzy, 1997; Asch, 1984). The social constructions that focus on deafness as a pathology (Kokaska, Woodward, & Tyler, 1984) obscure the importance of individual characteristics and overlook an understanding of deafness as a way of life (Leigh, 1999; Asch, 1984).

From a multicultural perspective, the positive identification of deaf individuals encompasses the integration of intrapsychic, social, familial, and cultural identification processes. Psychotherapists, anthropologists, and deaf individuals in the field consider some deaf individuals to be culturally Deaf, noting that individuals who have a different way of obtaining information (American Sign Language), and interpreting the world have an opportunity to share common socialization experiences in the Deaf world that results in a social identity (Parasnis, 1996; Padden, 1996; Corker, 1994; Higgins, 1983). These individuals also develop a different meaning to deafness than that of hearing mainstream society. Lane, Hoffmeister, and Bahan (1996) note, "Language has fundamentally three roles in bonding a group of speakers to one another and their culture. It is a symbol of social identity, a medium of social interaction, and a store of cultural knowledge. ASL (American Sign Language) fulfills all those roles in the culture of the Deaf-World" (p. 67).

Deaf and hard-of-hearing individuals vary in their acculturation and involvement in the Deaf world (Leigh, 1999). Body language, facial expressions, and visual movements are ways to communicate in the deaf world. Attendance at Deaf residential schools or involvement in the Deaf community promotes a strong identification process; this process incorporates values that are ego syntonic to deaf and hard of hearing individuals (Kannapell, 1993). The Deaf community provides opportunities for empowerment and self-actualization of its members, incorporating different values than hearing society. It is important to note that the sense of "hearing" is not valued as a means of identification, self-actualization, self-accomplishment, or a means to a rewarding life. Deaf culture values a group identification, group decision-making, and group mutual aid. "Deaf" values are part of the adaptation to an oppressive physical and social environment that stigmatizes deaf individuals. Deaf culture challenges the "hearing" perspective, that deafness is a deficit and that there is something wrong with deaf individuals. It augments a sense of self-respect and permits an individual to develop a sense of self-worth and dignity, challenging many of the stereotypical processes that one encounters in the hearing world.

It is important to note that the meaning of deafness, Deaf identity, and the process of acculturation or assimilation in the Deaf community are diverse among its members (Leigh, 1999). Communication styles are greatly impacted by the individual's age at the time of his/her hearing loss, as well as the type and degree of hearing loss. Ultimately the form of communication used such as manual communication (signed English, American Sign Language) or oral communication (lip-reading, speech) will greatly impact developmental, linguistic, cognitive, educational, psychological, familial and social processes (Higgins, 1983). Individuals who become deaf later in life, for example, have acquired spoken language skills and may be able to use residual hearing for speech reading. On the other hand, those who are born deaf or become deaf prior to the acquisition of language may rely on manual forms of communication such as American Sign Language or signed English. Individuals may consider themselves hard-of-hearing, deafened, orally deaf, Culturally Deaf, bicultural, or in fact do not feel their deafness is a significant factor in their identity.

STUDY

The study focused on understanding the special considerations necessary for effective treatment with deaf and hard-of-hearing individuals. The inductive nature of this project, grounded theory, attempted to break from a hearing model of values adopted by mainstream hearing society.

The investigator advertised at Gallaudet University, a liberal arts university for deaf and hard of hearing students. One e-mail announcement to the general Gallaudet population-staff, faculty, and students generated over ten responses. Flyers were distributed to dorms, recreational centers, and libraries on campus. All participants who were part of the actual study were college students at Gallaudet University. This is a significant factor, because Gallaudet University is the only liberal arts university for deaf individuals. The unique campus/community emphasizes the practice of sign language as the primary form of communication. Although Gallaudet University prides itself on acceptance of diversity, individuals who have various hearing losses, communication styles, and identity processes, all students must learn sign language as classes are conducted in signed communication.

Individuals who responded to the announcement and met all the requirements of the study were selected to be participants. Participants were deaf or hard-of-hearing, over the age of 18 years old, and had been in psychotherapy for at least several months within the past five years. Due to the diverse language levels of deaf and hard-of-hearing individuals, the sample population was limited to individuals who had some college education. A pilot study of seven individuals who were deaf or hard-of-hearing, faculty and students as well as individuals in the community, were interviewed. Upon revision of the methodology, ten participants were interviewed; 20% were participants of color, 20% were individuals raised in a foreign country, and 30% were males. Variation in the degree of hearing loss, communication styles, and meaning of deafness among the participants were noted.

Since many participants had multiple psychotherapy experiences, their most recent psychotherapy or the psychotherapy that was most significant to them received the most attention. In part, this decision was based on the results of the pilot study, which indicated that participants were most able to recall the recent or most powerful experiences.

DEVELOPMENT OF METHODOLOGY

The review of the literature in deafness and multiculturalism as well as the extensive clinical experience of the investigator identified several themes pertinent to the therapy process: competency in the field of deafness, lack of accessibility to mental health services, communication processes, the therapeutic relationship, and confidentiality. As previously stated, a pilot study was conducted to refine the methodology of the study. Initially the investigator asked open-ended questions about the participant's experiences in therapy. Many participants of the pilot study were not comfortable with the "unstructured nature" of the process; therefore the structure and order of the questions were changed. The researcher began with semi-structured, non-threatening questions in order to develop a rapport and initial comfort level during the interview. The change of structure of the interview process greatly enhanced the comfort level of the participants. Consultation from the Center on ASL Literacy resulted in the addition of prompt questions to help the participants understand the question and guide the explanation of experiences.

The review of the literature (Cannon, 1983; Gerber, 1983; Anderson & Rosten, 1985; Haley, 1988; Marschark, 1993; Bat-Chava, 1994; Clymer, 1995; Glickman, 1996; Lytle & Lewis, 1996; Harvey, 1999) and extensive experience of the researcher, consultation from the Center on ASL Literacy, and the pilot interviews helped develop the interview format. The following topics were included in the interviewing process: (a) accessibility to mental health services, (b) beneficial and negative experiences in psychotherapy, (c) relationship with the therapist, (d) implications of the hearing status of the therapist, (e) confidentiality issues, (f) recommendations for psychotherapists who work with deaf and hard-of-hearing individuals. Themes from the data were shaped by both the questions as well as the participants' stories of their experiences in psychotherapy.

Each participant answered a demographic questionnaire. One semi-structured interview with each participant was conducted. The researcher used visual modalities as a means of communicating and obtaining information; therefore, the interviews were video-taped. The investigator, who is deafened, acquired American Sign Language proficiency later in life; therefore, she received consultation in converting English-based questions to ASL. The investigator followed up on two interviews to assure accuracy of the videotape. All interviews were videotaped and transcribed from American Sign Language to English by an ASL transcriber (if ASL was the primary form of communication for the participant).

Bias and Limitations

Although intensive interviews uncovered many themes and processes related to psychotherapy for deaf and hard-of-hearing individuals, the pool of participants was limited. The study did not include, for example, any participant who had the cochlear implant or who had experienced an acute onset of hearing loss as an adult or older adult. Although the researcher tried to obtain diversity among the sample, only 20% were individuals of color and 30% were males. Most of the participants were young adults and there were no older individuals. Increasing the number of participants would make the data more comprehensive and possibly add more to the development of themes.

All researchers attempt to limit their potential bias; the subjectivity of analyzing and reporting data is well noted. The life experience of the researcher, who was deafened later in life, implies a strong affiliation and identification with the hearing world. Thus, one bias may be related to the fact that the researcher was not born deaf, nor is she integrally involved in the Deaf community.

A second bias relates to the fact that the participants were college students at Gallaudet University. As stated previously, Gallaudet University has its own political/social values and norms related to deafness. The sociopolitical climate within the Deaf world is changing to keep up with advances in technology and educational philosophies, thus the university is admitting more students who are hard-of-hearing or orally deaf. However, all courses are taught in sign language; therefore, the university supports a specific style of communication as well as way of coping with deafness. Although most of the participants were culturally Deaf and used ASL, several were oral or learning sign language. It is important to note, however, that this population does not represent the general pool of deaf individuals, who are mostly oral. The pool of participants excluded deaf individuals who were not educated. The clinical dynamics and communication processes for those individuals would obviously require an entirely different set of criteria and evaluation tools.

Data Analysis Procedures

The actual data analysis involved identifying and categorizing themes in the narrative data of each participant's interview. Initially these categories of themes and sub-themes were organized by gathering every response of each participant to each question, which was coded. Broad themes developed. After the responses were gathered, the researcher mapped and counted the number of respondents who commented on each theme. Finally, the researcher compared and contrasted responses in order to develop a composite picture of the variations (Anastas & McDonald, 1994).

Several factors contributed to the rigor and trustworthiness of this study. Interdisciplinary triangulation was practiced by including a deaf social worker, hearing researcher, anthropologist, and sociologist as consultants (Drisko, 1997). As stated previously, consultation was received at the Center on ASL Literacy to assist in the development of the interviewing tools. Debriefing sessions, "The process of exposing oneself to disinterested peer in a manner paralleling an analytic session for the purpose of exploring aspects of the inquiry that might otherwise remain only implicit within the inquirer's mind" (Lincoln & Guba, 1985, p. 308), was practiced as another method of establishing credibility. One deaf clinician offered to code portions of the transcript in order to compare and contrast the coding categories. This process helped the investigator begin to "distance" from the data in order to develop broad categories that were intertwined through the research.

For the purposes of this article, four major themes will be addressed: (a) cultural knowledge and sensitivity, (b) importance of communication processes, (c) the use of the social work/therapeutic relationship, (d) culturally syntonic interventions in work with deaf and hard of hearing individuals.

CULTURAL KNOWLEDGE

Basic tenets of multicultural literature emphasize the importance of understanding diverse values and norms of individuals from diverse cultural, social, and religious backgrounds (Lum, 1996). As Glickman (1996a) notes, "Culturally affirmative therapists value cultural differences as healthy expressions of human diversity and see connections between empowerment of a people, affirmation of their culture, and the individual mental health of the community's members" (p. 7). Results of this project note that social workers should understand the importance of and gain knowledge of deaf and hard of hearing identification processes, which includes multicultural identification, have knowledge of specific norms and values within social contexts, understand the importance of diverse communication styles, and understand the stigma of deafness and the ramifications of oppressive forces faced by deaf individuals and minority communities.

The social workers' understanding an individual's social Deaf identity plays a significant factor in the development of an individual's self esteem (Bat-Chava, 1994). Al, a participant of this study, clearly identified himself as bi-cultural, identifying with his paternal deaf grandfather as well as his hearing parents. The respondent struggled with an "overbearing" mother who made all the decisions for him. Al's problems were not related to deafness per se, but to familial processes. Al had a therapist who, unaware of Deaf identification processes, tried to convince him of the benefits of a cochlear implant. The therapist's lack of cultural knowledge and inaccurate assessment of Al's problems resulted in additional anxiety and self-doubt:

> When I was in _____ Hospital discussing the cochlear implant
> with _____ I obviously spoke negatively about it. He (therapist)
> didn't seem to believe me . . . he tried to convince me that there

was a newer procedure. Looking back I felt that he should not have tried to convince me because I was "not well" and a patient here. I felt he thought I was "not thinking straight" about the cochlear issue because I was not well.

Al's therapist was not cognizant of the importance of Al's cultural identification and affiliation with the Deaf community. However, an orally deaf client may desire the implant to enhance their functioning in the hearing world. Knowledge of cultural norms and values is essential in order to make appropriate assessments and interventions.

Norma's story emphasizes the understanding of diverse norms and values as it relates to various "deaf" settings. As a youngster, Norma transferred from a mainstream educational program to a school for the Deaf. Communication processes in the mainstream program focused on the use of spoken English whereas the Deaf school used American Sign Language as the primary mode of communication. The "use of English" and total communication signifies the value of integration into hearing society. ASL use, however, usually facilitates the social identification process of cultural Deafness. Thus, communication is a medium for socialization processes that allows the individual to gain self-understanding as well as internalize norms and values of the social environment. Linguistic development ultimately determines one's interpretation and understanding of the internal and external world. The form of communication used within a specific context greatly impacts on socialization processes and inherent values and norms. Norma, a beginning signer, used English word order when she entered the school for the deaf. Due to her communication style, her peer group ostracized her. Norma's deaf therapist understood her struggle to be accepted into this new environment:

> I was frustrated . . . first of all, it was my first "deaf experience"–a new environment. Deaf Culture, they signed ASL, while I signed English . . . They picked on me and made fun of my signs because I signed English. I tried to fit in.

Norma's experience emphasizes the importance of gaining knowledge of cultural values and norms for groups who are diverse.

From a social constructivist perspective, understanding the depth of oppression and stigma related to deafness is a component of cultural sensitivity. Selma, who felt she was different than others, struggled to understand her identity as a deaf woman. As an adolescent, her therapist did not understand the ramifications of her mother's negativism about deafness. Selma reported that she did not feel validated because her therapist tried to normalize her experience, but telling her that she was going through a normal adolescent experience:

> I do understand that the therapist may be right if it's related to puberty issues . . . teenagers trying to be independent of their parents . . . whether they are deaf or hearing . . . but I had specific problems with my deafness because my mother viewed my deafness as a medical issue . . . that there was something wrong with me and it needed to be fixed. I always knew that there was something wrong with that perspective . . . I always wanted to distance myself from my mother and not do things with her.

The above experience highlights the importance of familial processes that greatly impact on one's self esteem. Deaf individuals may internalize negative introjects about their deafness from significant others. Therefore, cultural knowledge includes an understanding of diverse identification processes, developmental challenges as well as values and norms of specific social/contexts (Mattei, 1996).

COMMUNICATION

The overriding theme emerging from this study is that of communication. Although participants had diverse styles of communication, from oral speech reading and use of voice to manual communication of American Sign Language, all participants noted the importance of communication processes. Communication is the foundation in which people understand each other. The use of signing, speech, body language, muscle tension, eye movement, facial gestures, pace and direction of movements, voice tones as well as the use of interpreters are all aspects of the communication process.

The communication challenge between deaf participants who did not have oral skills and hearing therapists who did not sign is noted. Jackie, a deaf participant, used ASL and struggled to be understood by her non-signing therapist. She was not used to using her voice and at times felt her voice was not intelligible:

> Awful . . . sometimes it was awful because when I'm talking about something emotional, I can't control my voice. If I'm speaking

with signs as well, I can't control my voice better. My voice tends to be lower when I'm emotional and the therapist can't hear nor understand me. When I get too emotional, I can't speak clearly . . . this means I have to suppress my emotions to speak clearly.

Marti's struggle to understand her therapist illustrated the differences in understanding the cultural meanings of communication styles between hearing and Deaf cultures. Individuals who have a hearing loss rely on their vision, their "seeing skills" to obtain information and communicate with others. Facial expressions are an important form of communication in the deaf world:

Maybe it's not that she didn't understand me, but she didn't have very strong reactions to what I said. She didn't say things like, "Oh yes, I understand . . ." I felt like the therapist (hearing therapist) did not understand because she would look at me with a poker face and sort of think, "Oh, that's your experience?"

Clearly, it is unrealistic to expect that social workers learn sign language or be proficient in ASL. However, understanding the basic tenets and struggles of communication can enhance the therapeutic process. Several participants suggested that the issues of communication be brought up during the initial sessions. In addition, the use of interpreters may alleviate some of the communication challenges that may occur. Ray, a deaf participant, reported improved communication with the use of an interpreter:

R: Boy, at the first session with her, I just nodded my head pretending that I understood her . . . so I got an interpreter.
I: How was it with an interpreter?
R: I liked it because I could understand better.

Although interpreters can greatly enhance the communication process, challenges can occur (Roe & Roe, 1991). One participant expressed concern about the interpretation of his feelings:

I felt I needed to work extra hard to show them who I am . . . what my feelings are . . . to share my feelings through English, I had to work harder . . . sign more in PSE (combination of ASL and English) order, use less body movements and facial expressions . . . it is energy draining . . . making sure the interpreter knows what I mean.

Another participant reported that it took longer to feel comfortable in the therapy session because of the presence of two individuals. In general, several participants recommended that more time be allotted to deal with the communication challenges that are encountered in the therapy sessions. One respondent noted, "We write back and forth. I decided to stop going . . . because it took too much time."

In addition to the mechanical aspects of understanding each other, social workers should be cognizant of the underlying clinical dynamics related to the experience of communicating. For most deaf individuals, communication processes may a core struggle in their life, the essence of deep-seated childhood experiences. Although social workers may not know how to sign, understanding the fact that communication struggles trigger transference, countertransference and may re-enact previously traumatic experiences is an important component of cultural sensitivity. Belinda, a deaf participant was seeing a hearing therapist who never worked with a deaf client. She discussed her experience:

> At first, I didn't think it would be a big deal, after a while, I realized I was always asking him to repeat himself. Sometimes the therapist would be "fed up" with that and would ask my mom, who was in the waiting room, to come and interpret for me (rolling eyes) . . . I couldn't tell the therapist everything because I didn't want my mom to know everything about my life. I would hold back some of the information. It was embarrassing because I was trying to be independent . . . It hurt because I thought he didn't want to deal with me and preferred to deal with hearing patients only.

Re-enactments and retraumatizations can be worked through with a sensitive therapist who is cognizant of the process. Empathic failures can lead to growth, if in fact the therapist is able to be aware of the process. Belinda's therapist was unaware of his countertransferential processes that reinforced feelings of low self-esteem on the part of Belinda.

DIFFERENTIAL USE OF SELF

Tenets of multicultural therapy focus on the importance of the therapeutic relationship (D'Ardenne & Mahtani, 1989; Durst, 1994). The "holding environment," a relationship between therapist and client, validates and supports the individual (Goldstein, 1995). The holding environment appears to be an essential component of treatment for those individuals who experience considerable oppression and stigma due to their deafness. This study raised an important question: Are social workers aware of the extent of the need for a holding environment for deaf clients? It appears that the consequences of oppression and internalization of negative introjects related to deafness necessitates a considerable amount of "holding," validating the individual's self worth and building on the individual's strengths. The importance of this validation, may at least initially transcend cross-cultural differences between clients and their therapists. Both Black participants who received therapy from white therapists reported tremendous satisfaction with their therapist, emphasizing the sensitivity to deafness. Although they reported that the cross-cultural issues were not significant, in part, these experiences may represent the depth of oppression and lack of resources for those individuals who are deaf.

Two thirds of the participants expressed concern about their parents' attitude towards their deafness. Several participants felt labeled as the problem in the family. One participant was adopted, another given up for guardianship to a deaf adult. Lena internalized a sense of "worthlessness" about herself from her mother. She stated, ". . . for years I felt that I did something wrong, but whatever, I realize it's not me, it's her (mother). It seems that she has issues but never went to a therapist." One respondent discusses her father's attitude towards her deafness, "He made me feel stupid . . . for years, I felt I did something wrong." The internalization of negative introjects internalized from parents or significant others may result in a very harsh super ego. Kim's story is a poignant example:

> I wondered if (it was) my fault that he (father) was an alcoholic because everyone in the family is hearing except for me and it's easy to be suspicious of that. It would have been a different story if there was another deaf member. The therapist helped me look at it from his perspective and taught me how alcoholism can be hereditary.

Seventy percent of the respondents who had hearing parents expressed concern about their parents' attitude towards their deafness. A significant percentage of respondents appeared to internalize the negative introjects related to being deaf. One respondent stated, "I remember having serious problems dealing with my deafness when I was a sophomore. I was feeling I was limited and it was difficult to cope with." Another respondent discussed her mother's attitude towards her deafness: "She made me feel stupid . . . for years, I felt I did something wrong." Thus the therapist's attitude towards deafness (Brauer, 1978; Harvey, 1989; Glickman, 1996a; Lane, Hoffmeister, & Bahan, 1996) may be the most significant factor in the therapeutic relationship. As one participant said, "My therapist helped me accept myself more." It is important to note that trans-cultural relationship can be effective, if the therapist has a positive attitude.

In addition to the importance of the positive regard of the therapist, early family intervention (Meadow-Orlans, 1987) may assist families in understanding and coping with their deaf child. The intervention process may facilitate grieving, challenge negative construction of deafness, and develop better communication strategies between deaf and hearing members.

The use of the relationship can provide opportunities for role modeling, positive identification of a deaf identity as well as internalization of values and norms that enhance one's self esteem (St. Claire, 1996). At the time of her therapy, Sally had a progressive hearing loss. She was a new signer who was not proficient in American Sign Language. Her therapist, however, was deaf and used American Sign Language as his primary mode of communication. The different communication styles presented challenges that Sally encountered in her world. Her therapist, however, was an effective role model in helping Sally become assertive and develop coping strategies to deal with her hearing loss:

> At first it was awkward, but later we developed our own method so when I couldn't understand him, he would write it down. If he couldn't understand me, then I would try again . . . we would work together on that. I should say that sometimes it was kind of an ESP because when I would think of something, he would then tell me not to think of that . . . then I would ask him what he thought I was thinking. We would joke about that.
>
> Through him, I learned not to be afraid to ask someone to repeat something if I didn't understand it. That was a difficult issue for me; for many years as I was always afraid to ask someone to repeat what they said if I didn't understand it. I had always let it go by me.

A strong therapeutic relationship may provide opportunities for positive identification between the therapist and client. Several participants developed a strong identification with their therapists. Melanie stated,

"I noted that I liked deaf therapists better than the hearing ones . . . sad to say. I think it has a lot to do with the bonding I feel with them." Robin's identification with her therapist was a powerful one. Robin, who lost her hearing, was seen by a therapist who had lost his hearing. She reported:

> He (therapist) also became deaf. The fact that he shared his experience with me helped me feel I could get over it and deal with what was going on in my life . . . The fact that he was deaf had an impact on my therapy because I looked at him as a role model . . . He was able to tell me that no matter what . . . no matter how much hearing I lost, I could deal with it.

The research supports the literature on multiculturalism reinforcing flexibility in the roles of therapist (Zitter, 1996). Glickman (1996a, p. 29) emphasizes role flexibility as, ". . . skills in expanding and flexing clinical roles and skills in collaboration with indigenous healers, helpers, community leaders, and paraprofessionals . . ." emphasizing the therapist's willingness to make home visits and be flexible about availability. Jerry appreciated the flexibility of this therapist:

> What the school psychologist did was take my brother and I to see my mother in the hospital so we can straighten out our issues. I really respected him for that . . . doing that outside his work.

Flexibility on the part of the therapist involved the extension of time allotted for treatment, willingness on the part of the therapist involved to make home visits and set up collateral meetings with significant others such as clergy; as well as make additional efforts to have the therapist accessible, and provide additional support and advocacy for client rights.

Over half the respondents noted the importance of sharing oneself in the process. The differential sharing of the therapist resulted in experiencing less isolation, validating the respondents' experiences, instilling a sense of hope and normalizing the experience. A poignant example is Dana's experience, "The fact that he (therapist) shared his experience helped me feel that I could get over it." Although social workers must be attuned to the possibility of increasing dependency, intensifying transferences, as well as diffusing boundary issues, the research supports the differential use of the therapist sharing of experiences when appropriate.

Therapists must be cognizant of the use of the therapeutic relationship with the treatment context. Clinical dynamics of transference, countertransference, re-enactments as well as the power of the corrective therapeutic experience can serve as a vehicle for social-emotional reeducation (Mattei, 1996; St. Claire, 1996). Although this project begins to address transcultural issues with the context of the deaf/hearing dyad, the most important aspect of the therapy process appears to be a culturally sensitive therapist who has a positive attitude related to hearing loss.

EGO/CULTURALLY SYNTONIC INTERVENTIONS

As previously stated, findings indicate that fundamental principles of effective interventions strategies for deaf and hard-of-hearing individuals entail the therapist's ability to be culturally sensitive which includes understanding the specific developmental challenges, clinical and mechanical dynamics of communication (Haley, 1989), the importance of experiential processes as well as the use of the therapeutic self as part of the corrective experience (Durst, 1994; Patterson, 1996; Harvey, 1998). Empowerment strategies such as encouragement, validation, education, challenging stereotypical processes, enhancing self-awareness, developing coping strategies and shifting responsibility to the client are essential components of effective therapy.

Are social workers aware of the extent of their need to develop an observing ego and self-awareness? Deaf individuals who are raised in linguistically inaccessible environments may have difficulty developing an understanding of themselves and others. Barbara, a deaf respondent who communicated via ASL, grew up in a hearing family with minimal communication. She stated that she never had a "mirror" growing up because of the barriers of communication with her parents. She described how the therapist helped her develop self-awareness and understanding of the impact of her behavior on others.

Deaf individuals who could not communicate with their families may have relied on visual and experiential processes to make sense of the world. This may be compounded by Corker's (1994) contention that forcing language (English) on deaf children may result in negativism and discomfort in expressing themselves in this modality. In addition, the experiences of silences and "passivity" may re-enact or have negative meaning to those individuals who great up in linguistically inaccessible environments. Several respondents stated that they desired an "active therapist." Although the meaning of active participation varied among the participants, most of them interpreted the therapist's active "listening" to signify passivity and at times disinterest: "I often talk, talk, talk, and the therapist listens, yet that can't do it for me." Another respondent stated, "I preferred to have an ongoing conversation when we take turns talking and just him listening all the time." A third respondent reported, "She didn't talk very much as she was expecting me to do all the talking . . . I didn't like that at all. I wanted her to talk too."

Findings suggest the use of non-verbal processes that include the use of experiential exercises are effective modalities in treatment. Nonverbal modalities are useful tools to access unconscious processes, develop self-awareness, and provide avenues for exploration. One participant noted: "If I get stuck at expressing my thoughts, she (therapist) would suggest that I draw or find another way to make it easier for me to express my feelings." Bob, another respondent, elaborated on the importance of aesthetics of the therapy office,

> The office I was in was very nice, warm . . . not just white walls with two chairs in it . . . a very nice environment and that's what I liked about it . . . Familiar things in the room helped me feel comfortable with my therapist.

CROSS CULTURAL ISSUES

The literature recognizes the complexity of discrimination for deaf Black individuals (Creamer, 2000). Creamer notes that due to racism and disenfranchisement, Black families have developed extended family network and kinship systems for support. She notes, "All the cultural, economic, and social circumstances that impact Black families also influence Black deaf families. It is noted that because of the negative experience with American society, Black parents may not seek social services or community support to help them with their deaf children. In addition, support services and community outreach programs may not be accessible. For example, Gallaudet University did not admit students of color until the 1950s. Therefore, clinicians need to be sensitive to multiple layers of discrimination.

An interesting finding in the study is that both Black deaf participants reported significant satisfaction with their white therapists because they felt their therapists were sensitive to the deaf issue. Although the investigator attempted to pursue the cross-cultural issues that surfaced in treatment, the participants did not readily discuss any issues. This may suggest that there are complicated transcultural processes that have not been identified, that some of the participants experienced multiple layers of discrimination, they did not feel "entitled" to discuss cross-cultural concern or in fact were not comfortable discussing the issue with a white investigator.

As stated in the previous section, the meaning of deafness may vary within diverse cultures and countries. One participant of a European country described the school for the hard-of-hearing as an institution that attempts to have children develop oral skills and integrate in a hearing society. She was unaware of the cultural identification process of deafness until her entrance into the United States as a young college student. She stated that she was not able to find one signing therapist in her country, thus feeling that most therapists were not accessible to her. Another participant from Jamaica described a life-time of trying to hide her deafness until she came to this country as a teenager. The above experiences strongly imply the importance of understanding the meaning of deafness, within both the cultural/social and psychological context. Those individuals from foreign countries did not have any exposure to Deaf culture or involvement in a Deaf community.

CONCLUSIONS

Individuals come to therapy for many different reasons. Although specific goals may vary, the focus of most treatment is to increase a client's sense of self worth and to empower his/her ability to function effectively in the world. The study suggests that deaf and hard-of-hearing individuals are challenged to find culturally sensitive social workers/therapists who can communicate effectively and understand their stories and their worlds. Although the processes and strategies discussed in this article are applicable to all populations, the importance and focus on these processes may be diverse. Social workers need to make accurate assessments of their clients; they must understand the meaning of deafness in a matrix that integrates the diverse influences, norms, and values that affect development and identity formation (Glickman, 1996b). This includes an understanding of intrapsychic and social stigma of deafness and specific developmental challenges that ultimately impact one's identity and self-esteem (Black, 1994). Social workers should integrate knowledge of social/psychological and cultural processes.

The study points to the importance of the relationship between social worker/therapist and client: unconditional acceptance. Corker (1994), in her discussion of methodological challenges in treatment, states, "the most important issue for me in choosing a counselor is for them to actually support me in my belief that there is nothing intrinsically wrong with me in terms of my deafness" (p. 125). Although unconditional acceptance is the most important/significant factor in the therapeutic relationship, understanding and clinical interventions related to the transcultural relationship (deaf/hearing) enhance the treatment process.

Culturally syntonic interventions emphasize the importance of empowerment processes for individuals who are at risk and who do not have access to the same information, power, or resources as others in their environment. Empowerment includes the imparting of information and education, advocacy, encouragement and reinforcement, development of self-awareness in order to develop appropriate coping mechanisms. A key component of treatment was the externalization of negative introjects from family of origin as well as from the social/cultural environment. In addition creative modalities of communication and self-expression may include non-verbal activities such as sports, art, psychodrama, and other experiential activities.

IMPLICATIONS FOR SOCIAL WORK EDUCATION

The basic tenets social work practice is applicable to work with deaf and hard-of-hearing populations. If possible, a course in disabilities would be recommended for students who are interested in working with deaf and hard-of-hearing populations. Parallel to courses in diversity, a specialized course in disabilities would sensitize students to the basic dynamics of individuals and populations that are disabled. Integration of curriculum content related to disabilities/deafness can be part of the HBSE, Policy, and Practice sequences.

Human Behavior and the Social Environment

The field of psycholinguistics is a new arena for social workers. The socialization and development of individuals who learn a different modality of communication has enormous significance as it relates to cognitive, linguistic, social, and psychological development. Historically deaf and hard-of-hearing people have experienced social and economic injustice. The native language of deaf individuals, American Sign Language, was denigrated and until recently forbidden in educational institutions. In addition to inaccessibility of mental health services, social, cultural and vocational programs, deaf and hard-of-hearing individuals have been subjected to discriminatory attitudes. Individuals with disabilities or those who are deaf or hard of hearing can be categorized in "populations at risk." An understanding of the oppression will help social workers apply principles of empowerment in their work with deaf and hard-of-hearing individuals.

Social workers should apply their knowledge of diversity to individuals/populations that are different. Parallel to multicultural tenets, deaf and hard of hearing individuals have diverse value systems, acculturation into deaf or hearing culture, diverse religious beliefs, socioeconomic backgrounds and cultural upbringing that impact on how one experiences oneself and the world. It is important for the culturally sensitive social worker to integrate their understanding of diversity in order to make accurate assessments, understanding of values, norms, human behavior, and experiences of deaf and hard of hearing individuals. Clearly it is impossible to impart information on all diverse groups; thus, this article emphasizes the importance of recognizing the need for continued self-learning related to diverse populations.

Social Work Practice

This research project attempts to begin to develop an awareness of the dynamics for individuals who have a hearing loss. The most prominent themes related to social work intervention include:

- effective communication and use of expressive modalities
- the importance of the experiential process of communication
- effective use of the therapeutic relationship with an emphasis on unconditional regard
- the importance of externalizing negative introjects related to deafness
- empowerment strategies
- development of ego syntonic interventions that emphasize the client's strengths
- Advocacy for accessible mental health services

Most social work interventions discussed in this article are applicable to all populations; however, the importance of these processes and the extent of use in the therapy session may be diverse. Social work practice incorporates an understanding of the unique challenges imposed by social/cultural/familial processes in the design of social work interventions.

Social Work Policy

The advent of ADA policies supported the empowerment of individuals who are disabled, including deaf and hard of hearing. From a macro perspective, community organizers need to assure a commitment from the community, social service agencies, and insurance companies to assign or identify and train therapists to work with this population. There are new programs that provide certificates in the field of deafness, including counseling, social work, and psychology. More recently, the development of a Commission on Disability within the Council of Social Work Education aims to sensitize social workers and social work students to the importance of understanding disability in the context of acquiring specific knowledge, skills, and sensitivity to diverse value systems.

Social work education can broaden the applicability of multicultural, symbolic interaction, social constructivist and empowerment paradigms that focus on sensitivity to diversity and differences to disabled populations.

REFERENCES

Anastas, J., & MacDonald, M. (1994). *Research design for social work and the human services*. NY: Lexington Books.

Anderson, G., & Rosten, E. (1985). Toward evaluating process variables in counseling deaf people: A cross cultural perspective. In D. Watson & G. Anderson (Eds.), *Counseling deaf people: Research and practice* (pp. 1-22). University of Arkansas: Arkansas Rehabilitation Research and Training Center on Deafness and Hearing Impairment.

Bat-Chava, Y. (1994). Group identification and self-esteem of deaf adults. *Personality and Social Psychology Bulletin, 20*, 494-502.

Black, R. (1994). Diversity and populations at risk: People with disabilities. In F. Reamer (Ed.), *Foundations of social work practice* (pp. 394-416). NY: Columbia University Press.

Brauer, B. (1978). Mental health and deaf persons: A status report. In *Gallaudet Today*, (fall), 9-13.

Bzuzy, S. (1997). Deconstructing disability: Impact of definition. *Journal of Poverty, 1*, 81-90.

Cannon, C. (1983). Use of interpreters in cross-cultural counseling. *The School Counselor, 31,* 11-18.

Clymer, E. (1995). The psychology of deafness: Enhancing self-concept in deaf and hearing-impaired. *Family Therapy, 22,* 113-120.

Corker, M. (1994). *Counselling: The deaf challenge.* Bristol, PA: Jessica Kingsley Publishers, Ltd.

Creamer, E. (2000). Deaf Black persons and their families: Ecological and systems perspectives. In *Journal of the American Deafness and Rehabilitation Association, 34,* 1-12.

D'Ardenne, P., & Mahtani, A. (1989). *Transcultural counseling in action.* NY: Sage Publications.

Drisko, J. (1997). Strengthening qualitative research studies and reports: Standards to promote academic integrity. *Journal of Social Work Education, 33,* 185-197.

Dubow, S., Geer, S., & Strauss, K. (1992). *Legal rights: The guide for deaf and hard of hearing people.* Washington, DC: Gallaudet University Press.

Durst, D. (1994). Understanding the client/social work relationship in a multicultural setting: Implications for practice. *Journal of Multicultural Social Work, 3,* 29-43.

Falicov, C. (1995). Training to think culturally: A multidimensional comparative framework. *Family Process, 34,* 373-388.

Gerber, B. (1983). A communication minority: Deaf people and mental health. *American Journal of Social Psychology, 3,* 50-57.

Glickman, N. (1996a). What is culturally affirmative psychotherapy? In N. Glickman & M. Harvey (Eds.), *Culturally affirmative psychotherapy with deaf individuals* (pp. 1-55). Mahwah, NJ: Lawrence Erlbaum Associates, Publishers.

Glickman, N. (1996b). The development of culturally Deaf identities. In N. Glickman & M. Harvey (Eds.), *Culturally affirmative psychotherapy with deaf individuals* (pp. 115-155). Mahwah, NJ: Lawrence Erlbaum Associated, Publishers.

Goldstein, E. (1995). *Ego psychology and social work practice.* NY: Free Press.

Haley, T.J. (1988). *Effects of similarity of disability and communication style on counselor social influence with deaf adolescents.* Unpublished doctoral dissertation, University of Nebraska, Lincoln.

Harvey, M. (1989). *Psychotherapy with deaf and hard of hearing persons: A systemic model,* Mahwah, NJ: Lawrence Erlbaum.

Higgins, P. (1983). *Outsiders in the hearing world: A sociology of deafness.* Beverely Hills, CA: Sage Publications, Inc.

Kannapell, B. (1993). *Language choice, identity choice: A sociolinguistic study of deaf college students.* Burtonsville, MD: Linstok Press.

Kokaska, C., Woodward, S., & Tyler, L. (1984). Disabled people in the Bible. *Rehabilitation Literature, 45,* 20-21.

Lane, H., Hoffmeister, R., & Bahan, B. (1996). *A journey into the Deaf-World.* San Diego, CA: DawnSignPress.

Leigh, I. (1999). Deaf therapists and the Deaf community: How the twain meet. In I. Leigh (Ed.), *Psychotherapy with deaf clients from diverse groups* (pp. 45-68). Washington, DC: Gallaudet University Press.

Lincoln, Y., & Guba, E. (1985). *Naturalist inquiry.* Newbury Park, CA: Sage Publications.

Lum, D. (1996). *Social work practice and people of color: A process stage approach.* Pacific Grove, CA: Brooks/Cole Publishers.

Lytle, L., & Lewis, J. (1996). Deaf therapists, deaf clients, and the therapeutic relationship. In N. Glickman & M. Harvey (Eds.), *Culturally affirmative psychotherapy with deaf persons* (pp. 261-279). Mahwah, NJ: Lawrence Erlbaum Associates, Publishers.

Marschark, M. (1993). Origins and interactions in social, cognitive, and language development of deaf children. In M. Marschark & D. Clark (Eds.), *Psychological perspectives on deafness* (pp. 7-24). Hillside, NJ: Lawrence Erlbaum Associates, Publishers.

Mattei, L. (1996). Coloring development: Race and culture in psychodynamic theories. In J. Berzoff, L. Melano, & P. Heertz (Eds.), *Inside out and outside in* (pp. 221-237). Northvale, NJ: Jason Aronson, Inc.

Meadow-Orlans, K.P. (1987). An analysis of the effectiveness of early intervention programs for hearing-impaired children. In M. Guralnick & F. Bennett (Eds.), *The effectiveness of early intervention programs for at-risk and handicapped children* (pp. 325-362). Orlando, FL: Academic Press, Inc.

Padden, C. (1996). From the cultural to the bicultural: The modern deaf community. In I. Parasnis (ed), *Cultural and language diversity and the deaf experience*. Cambridge, MA: Cambridge University Press.

Parasnis, I. (1996). *Cultural and language diversity and the deaf experience*. Cambridge, MA: Cambridge University Press.

Patterson, C. (1996). Multicultural counseling: From diversity to universality. *Journal of Counseling and Development, 74*, 227-231.

Roe, D., & Roe, C. (1991). The third party: Using interpreters for the deaf in counseling situations. *Journal of Mental Health Counseling, 13*, 91-105.

St. Clair, M. (1996). *Object relations and self psychology*. Monterey, CA: Brooks/Cole Publishing Company.

Steinberg, A., Sullivan, V.J., & Lowe, R. (1998). Cultural and linguistic barriers to mental health services: A deaf consumer's perspective. *The American Journal of Psychiatry, 155*, 982-984.

Steinberg, A., Sullivan, V. J., & Lowe, R. (1999). The diversity of consumer knowledge, attitudes, beliefs, and experiences: Recent findings. In I. Leigh (Ed.), *Psychotherapy with deaf clients from diverse groups* (pp. 23-44). Washington, DC: Gallaudet University.

Sussman, A., & Brauer, B. (1999). On being a psychotherapist with deaf clients. In I. Leigh (Ed.). *Psychotherapy with deaf clients from diverse groups* (pp. 3-22). Washington, DC: Gallaudet University.

Vernon, M. (1995). A historical perspective on psychology and deafness. *Journal of the American Deafness and Rehabilitation Association, 29*, 8-13.

Zitter, S. (1996). Report from the front lines: Balancing multiple roles of a deaf therapist. In N. Glickman & M. Harvey (Eds.), *Culturally affirmative psychotherapy with deaf persons* (pp. 185-247). Hillsdale, NJ: Lawrence Erlbaum Associates, Publishers.

APPENDIX
Demographic Information

	Characteristic	Responses
Self Identification	Deaf	7
	Hard of Hearing	3
Deafness in Family	Parents	1
	Grandparents	2
	Siblings	1
Primary Mode	ASL	5
of Communication	English	2
	Bilingual (oral and manual)	2
	SimCom (voice and sign)	1
School Settings*	Mainstream	8
	School for the Deaf	8
	Deaf class in public school	5
	Private school for hearing children	1
	Public school–no assistance	1

* Adds up to more than 10 because some participants had multiple answers

Life Participation Approaches to Aphasia: International Perspectives on Communication Rehabilitation

Larry Boles
Mimi Lewis

SUMMARY. This paper discusses a recent development in aphasia treatment, termed the Life Participation Approach to Aphasia (LPAA) (Chapey et al., 2001). LPAA is a model of aphasia rehabilitation that is being practiced internationally in Canada, Australia, England, and the United States. This approach is consumer-driven, and emphasizes re-engagement in life. LPAA views family members and the larger community as active contributors to the rehabilitation process. Rather than focusing on the hypothetical situations depicted in pictures, real-life social interactions comprise the therapy context with LPAA. *[Article copies available for a fee from The Haworth Document Delivery Service: 1-800-HAWORTH. E-mail address: <docdelivery@haworthpress.com> Website: <http://www.HaworthPress.com> © 2003 by The Haworth Press, Inc. All rights reserved.]*

Larry Boles is Associate Professor, Department of Speech Pathology & Audiology, California State University-Sacramento, Sacramento, CA 95819.

Mimi Lewis, DCSW, LCSW, CSAC, is Faculty Lecturer, Division of Social Work, California State University-Sacramento, Sacramento, CA 95819.

[Haworth co-indexing entry note]: "Life Participation Approaches to Aphasia: International Perspectives on Communication Rehabilitation." Boles, Larry, and Mimi Lewis. Co-published simultaneously in *Journal of Social Work in Disability & Rehabilitation* (The Haworth Press, Inc.) Vol. 2, No. 2/3, 2003, pp. 47-64; and: *International Perspectives on Disability Services: The Same But Different* (ed: Francis K. O. Yuen) The Haworth Press, Inc., 2003, pp. 47-64. Single or multiple copies of this article are available for a fee from The Haworth Document Delivery Service [1-800-HAWORTH, 9:00 a.m. - 5:00 p.m. (EST). E-mail address: docdelivery@haworthpress.com].

KEYWORDS. Aphasia, treatment, social, "quality of life," international, interdisciplinary, "social work," "speech pathology," "speech therapy," "life participation"

INTRODUCTION

Aphasia is an acquired communication disorder that is caused by brain damage (Chapey & Hallowell, 2001). In most cases, speaking, writing, reading, and comprehension of the spoken word are all impaired to some degree (Parr, Byng, & Gilpin, 1997). Stroke (also known as "cerebral vascular accident" or CVA) is the most common cause of aphasia, although brain tumors and traumatic brain injury can also bring about the disorder. Aphasia has a range of types and severity, but in every case the difficulty of retrieving words is affected (Brookshire, 1997). The elderly are most at risk for stroke, thus for aphasia. Two-thirds of all strokes occur in people over the age of 65, and the risk of stroke doubles each decade after the age of 55 (National Stroke Association, 2001). If an individual with aphasia wishes to discuss a trip to the grocery store, the description could (in one type of aphasia) sound like the following:

> Client: um, store [gestures steering car] and nan-um ba-nan-a and hmm, not here, not in store. So me uh "hey sir, um where um [gestures peeling of banana]," and he uh "What?" so I uh "well, not apple, not that there, but [gestures peeling banana again]" and he "oh yeah!" and later 1-2-3 [points to watch] 5 times and ba-nan-a.

Treatment for aphasia invariably includes a regimen of speech-language therapy. Most of the speech-language approaches involve didactic interaction between the therapist and client, without regard to the naturally occurring environments in which the client might interact. These approaches focus on the client's ability to utter words. Using the above example, a traditional approach to aphasia treatment would pursue the utterance of the message "there are no bananas here," rather than focusing on reinforcing the client's social contact with the produce worker or the success in requesting help in a public place.

This paper discusses a recent development in aphasia treatment, termed the Life Participation Approach to Aphasia (LPAA) (Chapey et al., 2001). LPAA is a model of aphasia rehabilitation that is being practiced internationally in Canada, Australia, England, and the United

States. This approach is consumer-driven, and emphasizes re-engagement in life. The focus of LPAA is thus broader than the utterance or language-level goals of traditional aphasia therapy (Vickers, 2003). LPAA is more flexible than the latter methods, and views family members and the larger community as active contributors to the rehabilitation process. Whereas traditional approaches often incorporate flashcards and workbooks, LPAA approaches tend to focus on situations within the patient's environment, including the significant others' participation. Rather than focusing on the hypothetical situations depicted in pictures, real-life social interactions comprise the therapy context with LPAA.

The proponents of LPAA are concerned with the complex relationships between the client's internal self, which has had to be redefined because of the disability of aphasia, and his or her external world (interpersonal relationships, community, physical environment) and how all of these entities influence each other over time. This particular focus of LPAA is reminiscent of social work's ecosystems perspective—the profession's leading approach or "metatheory" since the 1970s (Pillari, 2002). LPAA embraces the ecosystems perspective's concept of interactionism (Van Wormer, 1997), wherein the focus of treatment is the reciprocal exchange between the person with aphasia and the people and systems in his or her environment. Further, the series of changes being sought by the speech-language pathologists come as much from the non-aphasic individuals and systems as they do from the individual who has aphasia.

The purpose of this paper is to discuss each of the interventions within the LPAA model. Implications for social workers will also be discussed. Because this approach highlights families and systems relationships, this paper will close with a discussion about the potential for collaborative work with social workers. Before addressing each of the approaches within LPAA, a brief historical perspective will help shed light on this topic.

HISTORY OF APHASIA TREATMENT

Aphasia therapy originated from a disease model (Lyon & Shadden, 2001). The emphasis was on measuring and treating the symptoms—the linguistic shortcomings of the individual, and on "curing" the disease—the elimination or lessening of the symptoms. Although thousands of clients benefited from this approach, the effects on the person's communication outside the therapy room were not a concern. The clinical research of the 1970s and 1980s turned to the generalization of the treatment benefits to untreated conditions. This coincided with more sophisticated efficacy research designs (Kearns, 1989). The rigor of these experimental designs demanded that the gains made by individuals with aphasia be expanded beyond therapy walls. While scientifically sound, much of the research at this time was conducted by clinicians. As clinicians, they realized that clients were making changes in other aspects of communication beyond grammatical utterances.

Later in the 1980s clinical research began investigating alternative forms of communication, and more natural communicative contexts (Lyon & Shadden, 2001). Davis and Wilcox (1985) encouraged clinicians to accept communication beyond linguistic constraints, to include the use of gestures, drawing, and writing. Others began developing discourse methodologies (Bottenberg, Lemme, & Hedberg, 1987).

Although therapy gains for individuals were demonstrated (Wertz et al., 1986), strategies used in the clinic were not necessarily being used when clients spoke to their spouses or family members (Simmons, 1993). Boles (1998a) discussed the problem of having the primary stakeholders in communication sitting in the waiting room, while the medical-model-driven speech pathologist attempted to "fix the problem" in the therapy room. Simmons-Mackie and Damico (1997) noted that all parties involved in communicating with the individual with aphasia needed to have their communicative styles and needs considered.

In 1980 the World Health Organization established a taxonomy for chronic dysfunction (WHO, 1980), which was later updated such that consequences to disease were relegated to one of three levels: (a) the body (impairment); (b) the person (disability); and (c) the person as a social being (handicap) (Worrall, 2000). This taxonomy helped clinical researchers understand aphasia in a new framework. Much of the early research had focused on impairment-level recovery, with little or no regard to the person or the person as a social being. Recent clinical advances in aphasia have incorporated this view into aphasia therapy (Boles, 1997, 1998a, 1998b, 1999, 2000; Elman & Bernstein-Ellis, 1999; Kagan, 1998; Lyon, 2000; Simmons-Mackie, 2000). Chapey et al. (2001) defined an approach to aphasia described as "consumer driven," and that supported both immediate and longer term life goals of individuals with aphasia and others affected by it. This Life Participation Approach to Aphasia (LPAA) has gained international attention, and will be the topic of the remainder of this paper.

LIFE PARTICIPATION APPROACHES TO APHASIA

LPAA has at its core the strengthening of participation in activities of choice by the person with aphasia. This changes the entire focus of therapy from improving the verbal output of the individual to examining the entire communicative environment. The client now has a voice in all aspects of therapy, including therapy tasks and outcome measures. The responsibilities of therapists include addressing the client's environment–the people, situations, and support involved with communication. The following are the core values of LPAA as outlined by its proponents (Chapey et al., 2001):

1. The explicit goal is enhancement of life participation. In this regard, communication becomes a means to an end. The speech-language pathologist assesses not just the aphasia (i.e., comprehension of the spoken word, word retrieval, and so on), but the extent to which the aphasia affects the person's achievement of life participation goals.
2. All those affected by aphasia are entitled to service. Communication does not occur in a vacuum. Treating an aphasic individual without including a communication partner is equivalent to teaching a deaf individual sign language without including others in his or her environment. LPAA may include (but needn't be limited to) the inclusion of family members, friends, and/or other aphasic individuals–anyone who is considered a part of the individual's communication community.
3. The measures of success include documented life enhancement changes. The outcome measures include not only standardized communication assessments but life satisfaction measures (e.g., Chubon, 1987; Larsen, Diener, & Emmons, 1985), measures of psychosocial well-being and social participation (e.g., Bradburn, 1969; Lyon et al., 1997; Simmons-Mackie & Damico, 2001), and life-activities indices (Simmons-Mackie & Damico, 1996).
4. Both personal and environmental factors are targets of intervention. Personal factors have long been intervention targets. However, environmental targets for communication are analogous to providing ramps for wheelchair users. Kagan and Gailey (1993) advocate the provision of "communication ramps." These authors suggest that others assume some of the communication burden–again the analogy of having communication partners learn sign language applies. Communication with non-aphasic individ-

uals does not necessarily provide a good model for communicating with aphasic individuals. Speech-language pathologists (and their clients) learn early in their practice that certain strategies are quite beneficial (e.g., reducing speaking rate, using drawing, and gestures), although the effectiveness of strategies varies across patients.

5. Emphasis is on availability of services as needed at all stages of aphasia. Aphasia is a lifelong condition. The effects of aphasia on life participation may not be immediately felt. Then too, one's life circumstances evolve. There needs to be some awareness of the developmental changes of the individual. LPAA acknowledges that these changes should be addressed regardless of time post-onset.

LPAA IMPLEMENTATION INTERNATIONALLY

Clinical researchers in Canada, Australia, England, and the United States have applied LPAA to treatment, although each of the studies reviewed in this paper has a different configuration. The remainder of this paper describes these various manifestations of LPAA.

Canada

Supported Conversation

Kagan (1998) trains aphasic communities in Ontario, Canada. Her clients are often not individuals with aphasia, but the people who interact with them, in what she terms "Supported Conversation." Her clientele include friends and family members, physicians, nurses, speech-language pathologists, occupational therapists, and others who wish to converse more effectively with aphasic individuals. In Supported Conversation, volunteers are taught how to interact in a facilitative way with individuals with aphasia. Kagan uses the analogy of a "communication ramp," which can best be provided by volunteers educated in how to talk to a person with aphasia.

Kagan conducted a study to determine the efficacy of her methods of training volunteers (Kagan, Black, Duchan, Simmons-Mackie, & Square, 2001). Two key dependent measures were acknowledging (communicative) competence and revealing (communicative) competence. In the former measure, a conversational partner is talking in a natural manner, yet is sensitive to his or her communicative partner. Thus, unclear responses are handled respectfully, without patronization, and the conversational partner takes on a "listening attitude." With the second dependent measure, a partner *reveals* competence by ensuring the partner with aphasia understands (e.g., by using gesture, writing or drawing, or reacting to facial cues), by ensuring the partner with aphasia has a means of responding (e.g., by providing written choices, encourages drawing by the partner with aphasia), and by verifying what the partner with aphasia has said (verbally and nonverbally). The expected result of this research was that trained volunteers would perform significantly higher than untrained volunteers in both acknowledging and revealing competence after the one-day training (followed by 1.5 hours of hands-on practice). More remarkable than the improvement by trained volunteers was that individuals with aphasia who had interacted with trained volunteers increased on ratings of social and message exchange skills, even though they did not participate in the training. This improvement was not present in those who had interacted with untrained (i.e., control group) volunteers.

United States

Group Treatment Using LPAA

Roberta Elman and her colleagues include individuals with aphasia and any person expressing a desire to communicate with them in their communication groups. Clients have a large voice in therapy activities in the not-for-profit organization, Aphasia Center of California. Elman has reported success using group treatment paradigms with aphasic individuals (Elman & Bernstein-Ellis, 1999) in Oakland, California. All participants in this efficacy study were described as "chronically aphasic"–were more than six months post-onset of aphasia. Rather than grapple with the ethical issue of a non-treatment group, Elman and Bernstein-Ellis randomly assigned participants to immediate-treatment and deferred-treatment groups.

Therapy sessions (five hours per week for four months) were conversational in nature, and the topics were typically chosen by the individuals with aphasia rather than by the professionals. The speech-language pathologists served as facilitators rather than directors of conversation. The deferred-treatment group initially participated in movement groups, performance groups, and a support group. The immediate-therapy group scored significantly higher on linguistic and functional communication measures compared to pre-test measures, and significantly higher than the deferred treatment group. The deferred treatment group nonetheless benefited when they eventually received treatment, and scored as well as the immediate treatment group after their four-month therapy regimen. These effects were also present after a month of no treatment.

Communication Partners

Jon Lyon was one of the earliest advocates for including communication partners in helping people with aphasia. Lyon, however, went well beyond the traditional boundaries of aphasia treatment. For example, he recruited community volunteers to engage in activities chosen by the person with aphasia. These activities included gardening, traveling to nearby places, taking an art class, and walking dogs at the Humane Society. In a study examining the effects of this treatment (Lyon et al., 1997), 10 treatment dyads engaged in pre-treatment testing, five months of treatment, and follow-up testing. The treatment was divided into six weeks of functional communication training and 14 weeks of the above-mentioned activities, twice weekly. The study participants were all more than one year post-stroke (mean of 43 months).

As expected, no changes were noted in standardized communication measures. However, improvement was noted on measures of psycho-social well-being and communication readiness. Further, nine of the ten dyads continued participating in the activities chosen for the study in the months following the study, and eight of those dyads added activities in the subsequent months.

Social Approaches to Aphasia

Simmons-Mackie and Damico (2001) described a program designed for their client, "Karen," a schoolteacher prior to her stroke, who had reached a "plateau" with conventional therapy methods. This plateau was defined as a lack of improvement on standardized aphasia test batteries. Prior treatment had focused on the impairment to Karen (in the language of WHO, the "body" level). Little attention had apparently been devoted to the communication contexts to which Karen would return (i.e., the "person"). The clinician helped Karen develop a "contextual inventory of key life activities," which compared her pre-aphasia activities to those after aphasia onset. What emerged was a relatively impoverished social life following her stroke.

For Karen, at that time in her recovery, continuing work at the impairment level was analogous (once again) to increasing the vocabulary of a sign language learner, rather than providing opportunities for using the core vocabulary already learned. This client was encouraged to volunteer at a local preschool. The workers at the preschool were educated regarding facilitative acts to help Karen communicatively. Other outcomes included an adjustment from cooking her family's dinner (pre-aphasia) to hosting a family potluck (post-aphasia), and from functioning as the secretary of her club to being an attendee at her club.

The qualitative measures used to document Karen's improvement clearly showed a richer social network, increases in the contextual inventory of key life activities, and self-reports of improved self-esteem and independence. These self-reports were verified by many of the people in Karen's communicative network, lending credibility to the outcome reports.

Solution Focused Aphasia Therapy

Boles and Lewis (2000) originally used the solution focused approach with marriage therapy with a couple with aphasia and later adapted it for use in communication therapy (Boles & Lewis, 2001). The LPAA does not make a sharp distinction between "communication therapy" and couples' counseling therapy, however, and the distinction is more one of application of particular techniques than a philosophical distinction.

Solution focused therapy has its origins in social work (DeShazer, 1997), and uses the following principles:

1. The emphasis is not on a client's or client-system's problems, but rather on the "exceptions to the problems or problem behaviors." This distinction becomes poignant with aphasia, where communication traditionally seen as the "problem." With exceptions as the focus, the attention is turned to those times when communication (between the person with aphasia and the communication partner) is successful, rather than instances of failed communication. Analysis of successful communication occurs during therapy, in order to simulate or recreate those circumstances. For example, a successful communication interaction may have occurred between a married couple in the morning with relative quiet in the house, and the topic may have been a movie that the couple had seen the evening before. A "homework assignment" from a solution focused aphasia therapist might be for the couple to engage in

conversations in the morning, and to keep the topic on events of the previous 24 hours.
2. Emphasizing the positive. This idea is not unique to solution focused aphasia therapy, of course. However, coupled with exception-finding, the following dialog becomes common:

Him: It's been frustrating; she doesn't seem to understand me.
Therapist: When she does understand you, what does that look like? How do you know she understands (finding exceptions)?
Him: Well, she's looking at me, and maybe nods sometimes.
Therapist: How many times has she done that, say, in the last day?
Him: Gosh, I don't know maybe twice.
Her: No (holding up six fingers).
Therapist: Ah, six times. Fantastic. And that would make seven now, since you obviously understood that (emphasizing positive)!

3. Treatment goals are client-generated and realistic. These goals are outcome-oriented. That is, the therapist asks what the clients (both the person with aphasia and the communication partner–often the spouse) would like by the end of therapy. This is not unique to solution focused aphasia therapy (SFAT); however, the exception-finding once again points the couple in the direction of a solution. That is, the therapist will not help the couple explore the barriers to achieving that goal, but will instead help them examine those times when that goal was the closest to being realized. Scaled questions are often used for these goals, wherein the client is asked to rate his or her current level of the desired outcome on a scale of 1-10. The therapist urges the client to select a desired level for the goal on that same scale, to be a therapy target.

Beyond the above principles, the routine of SFAT involves short (3-5 minutes) in-session conversations, followed by check-ins by the therapist, wherein he or she gives feedback regarding the conversation. This feedback usually includes observations regarding one or more of the couple's stated goals, and always involves observations regarding what each of the participants did particularly well (i.e., emphasizing the positive). Sessions are thus conversational in nature, and needn't involve any of the typical therapy "materials" such as pictures or workbook exercises. Sessions more closely resemble counseling sessions, wherein the topic could be last night's conflict, sexual intimacy, or the grief associated with the disability.

Using this method, Boles (2000) reported success with a couple using SFAT. A man with moderate non-fluent aphasia of four years' duration improved on eight of 10 self-rated goals, while his wife improved on seven of 10. Minimal improvement was realized on a test for aphasia severity, but improvement judged to be clinically significant was realized on a functional assessment of communication. Facilitative gestures were slightly more frequent by the client and dramatically more frequent by his wife at the end of the four weeks of therapy.

For Boles' couple, like most methods reported in this paper, improvement was realized in the areas most important to the individuals in therapy, without change in traditional aphasia test scores. Boles suggests that the latter tests may not measure those skills that matter to the clients.

England

Autobiography as Method

Pound, Parr, and Duchan (2001) reported several cases wherein in-depth interviews guided the delivery and evaluation of services. Pound et al. interviewed the women whose husbands had acquired aphasia. These interviews resulted in therapy plans tailored to the specific needs of each couple. The rationale was: (a) aphasia affects not only the lives of those with aphasia, but their family members as well; (b) autobiographical accounts were inherently relevant to the individual clients; (c) as heterogeneous as aphasia can be, the impact on individuals is all the more diverse; and (d) the ongoing autobiographical descriptions offered a direct window into the impact of treatment on these clients.

On several accounts, the study by Pound and colleagues is in sharp contrast to traditional therapy and is unique among LPAA approaches as well. First, the therapy itself comprised provision of information, group discussion, and group activities. The latter activities comprised what many would consider "support group" activities. Second, the therapy involved the wives of the individuals with aphasia, rather than the individuals with aphasia, who are traditionally considered "the clients." Finally, the measures of success were geared toward the spouses as well, underscoring the LPAA core value that all those affected by aphasia are entitled to services.

Drawing

Sacchett, Byng, Marshall, and Pound (1999) described a therapy program used with people with severe aphasia. They used drawing as a medium to enable these individuals to converse with their caregivers. As they expected, the study participants improved in measures of drawing accuracy and recognizability, but not on measures of language. Follow-up interviews with caregivers revealed improved communication in the home. The study participants used by Sacchett and colleagues were all one year or more post-onset of aphasia, and were judged severely impaired communicatively.

Australia

Speaking Out

Worrall and Yiu (2000) used a group experimental design to determine the effects of volunteer-administered in-home therapy for 14 individuals with chronic aphasia. Volunteers provided 10 scripted modules (termed "Speaking Out") for the therapy portion of the study, using current adult learning theory in the design of the modules. After pre-treatment testing, Group A received the 10 week Speaking Out regimen, whereas Group B received 10 weeks of recreational activities. After 10 weeks of no therapy (withdrawal phase) in both groups, a 10-week regimen of recreational activities was administered to Group A, and 10 weeks of Speaking Out to Group B. Significant pre-test/post-test differences were found in both groups on tests of aphasia severity and on an activity/disability measure. Minimal differences were found between groups.

DISCUSSION

Life Participation Approaches to Aphasia have changed the focus of therapy in the global community. Not all the above method identify themselves as LPAA approaches, yet all adhere to its core values. This section discusses those values in relation to each of the methods reviewed.

Life Participation as a Goal

Lyon and colleagues' (1997) Communication Partners and Simmons-Mackie and Damico's (1997, 2001) social approach are perhaps the best examples of this value. Activities are chosen by the individual with aphasia, thereby facilitating empowerment by a person with at least one year of extreme struggle. Further, the person with aphasia is building (or rebuilding) a social interaction between himself or herself and a committed communication partner. This can then be used as a model for further social relationships. Finally, the activities provide a natural (what Simmons-Mackie and Damico, in 1996, called *authentic*) context within which the person with aphasia can use the skills learned in the first phase. This context is almost certainly more authentic than the traditional speech therapy office.

In the Social Approach of Simmons-Mackie and Damico, the client had been discharged from traditional impairment-focused therapy. Rather than dwell on the client's remaining impairment, these researcher-clinicians posed the question, "given the aphasia as a condition which will remain for the foreseeable future, how can we help this person?" Attention is then devoted to the contexts in which the client would use any improved skills, rather than on the skills themselves.

Elman and colleagues relinquished control of the activities, asking clients what they would like to do during the group therapy. The choice of activity did have a decidedly clinical focus; however, offering choices certainly increased the empowerment by the clients. The work of Boles (2000), Boles and Lewis (2000, 2001), Pound et al. (2001), Sacchett et al. (1999), and Worrall and Yiu (2000) are all aimed toward a more fulfilling participation in life, rather than improved communication skills at the "micro" level.

All Those Affected by Aphasia Are Entitled to Service

All the approaches reviewed for this paper utilize or otherwise offer services to others besides those with aphasia. In the extreme case, Pound and colleagues work only with the spouses of the people with aphasia. In Kagan's Supported Conversation, the attention is clearly on the volunteers working with the aphasic clients. This attention is somewhat more evenly divided between the two parties in Solution Focused Aphasia Therapy, the drawing therapy of Sacchett and colleagues, the social approach of Simmons-Mackie and Damico, Communication Partners and Speaking Out. In the latter five cases, dyads are the focus.

Measures of Success Include Documented Life Enhancement Changes

Each of the methods reviewed included some measure of life enhancement changes beyond the standardized aphasia batteries commonly reported in the literature. This is an important feature for any life participation approach, as the assumption of these approaches is that the person with aphasia will embark on a quest for life participation in the presence of a life-long aphasia. A reduction of the severity of aphasia is not the goal–rather it is the improvement in life participation. Thus, the measures of improvement must follow suit.

Both Personal and Environmental Factors Are Targets of Intervention

Some of the methods reviewed here address this issue more directly than others. Kagan's Supported Conversation and Pound and colleagues' work with the communication partners of those with aphasia. These partners could be viewed as a part of the aphasic individuals' environment. Lyon and colleagues, in Communication Partners, encouraged the dyads to modify any communicative environmental barriers possible. The same could be said for each of the other methods, although not necessarily explicitly stated.

Emphasis Is on Availability of Services As Needed at All Stages of Aphasia

All the approaches reviewed in this paper included only clients who had acquired aphasia one year or more prior to the study. Yet, the nations included in this paper have a pattern of providing services for the first weeks to months post-onset of stroke. There are at least two reasons that the clinical scientists include only "chronically aphasic" clients. First is a pragmatic/scientific one. The phenomenon of "spontaneous recovery" (Benson & Ardila, 1996) is widely accepted as a span of 6-12 months post-onset, wherein the swelling of the brain diminishes, and some of the neurons that were spared from the stroke begin to function more efficiently. The second reason for including chronically aphasic clients only is a political one–although services to chronically aphasic individuals has occurred, few speech pathologists and fewer clients with aphasia and their families believe that no benefit can be realized beyond the 6-12-month window. The pattern in the studies reviewed here was consistent–no progress on traditional measures of speech and language, but clear improvement on measures of functional communication and well-being.

IMPLICATIONS FOR SOCIAL WORK

Conspicuously absent from many of the LPAA approaches discussed has been the formal involvement of a social worker. Although two of the approaches (Boles & Lewis, 2001; Kagan, 1998) directly involve social workers, the fact remains that much of the LPAA model sounds as much like social work as it does speech-language therapy. How then, could social workers participate in LPAA approaches?

Case management and interdisciplinary team planning are roles familiar to nearly all hospital and outpatient social workers. The need for this case management is not eliminated when the client is discharged from the hospital, however. Often clients require additional social services, such as disability benefits, medical insurance coverage, respite care for caregivers, public transportation, durable medical equipment, and so on.

Co-treatment with speech-language pathologists has been reported (Boles & Lewis, 2000, 2001). Direct therapy with an emphasis on communication is a concept familiar to both speech-language pathologists and social workers. Social workers receive a good deal more training in group facilitation than speech-language pathologists, and could be useful as a team member for those approaches that incorporate groups.

Two of the LPAA approaches included community volunteerism. Social workers have a wealth of knowledge in community work and would be an asset to those efforts.

Finally, the social worker is well-qualified to participate in crisis intervention. It is not unusual for a stroke survivor to lose his or her job, with a detrimental effect on couple interaction, social contact, employment, and income. This combination of factors puts the individual with aphasia at high risk for the need for crisis intervention.

CONCLUSIONS

The evidence gathered for the effectiveness of LPAA thus far is encouraging. The fact that at least four countries have reported success using LPAA is also encouraging. These methods have been discussed in contrast to "traditional" methods (Chapey et al., 2001). Whether they establish their own tradition will require further evidence regarding efficacy.

The nature of the evidence for efficacy of LPAA must differ from the evidence of more traditional methods, however. Dependent variables for more traditional methods have typically comprised linguistic structures, length of utterances, and the ability to follow auditory commands. The result of using these variables has been demonstration of improved linguistic performance, increased length of utterance, and increased performance of auditory commands. These measures are useful to the scientist, and perhaps useful as means-to-ends for clients, but are only marginally important for life participation.

Given a preponderance of evidence supporting the efficacy of LPAA, what is the appropriate course? It appears that the life participation approaches discussed here lie at one end of the rehabilitation continuum, chronologically. It may be that the more traditional approaches are better suited for immediately acute stages of recovery, while LPAA are better suited for the chronically aphasic. On the other hand, why would a client want to wait for months after a stroke before addressing life participation? Further evidence is currently being gathered by many scientists to document the place of LPAA in the lives of those with aphasia.

REFERENCES

Benson, D., & Ardila, A. (1996). *Aphasia: A clinical perspective.* New York: Oxford University Press, p. 352.

Boles, L. (1997). Conversation analysis as a dependent measure in communication therapy with four individuals with aphasia. *Asia Pacific Journal of Speech, Language, and Hearing, 2,* 43-61.

Boles, L. (1998a). Conducting conversation: A case study using the spouse in aphasia treatment. Neurophysiology and Neurogenic Speech and Language Disorders: Special Interest Division Two Newsletter. *American Speech-Language-Hearing Association,* 24-31.

Boles, L. (1998b). Conversation analysis as a method for evaluating progress in aphasia: A case report. *Journal of Communication Disorders, 31,* 261-274.

Boles, L. (2000). Solution-Focused Aphasia Therapy. *CSHA,* November, 8-12.

Boles, L., & Lewis, M. (2000). Solution-focused co-therapy for a couple with aphasia. *Asia Pacific Journal of Speech, Language and Hearing, 5,* 73-78.

Boles, L., & Lewis, M. (2001). Solution focused aphasia therapy: A social approach. Mini-seminar, *American Speech-Language-Hearing Convention,* New Orleans, Louisiana, November 16, 2001.

Bottenberg, D., Lemme, M., & Hedberg, N. (1987). Effect of story content on narrative discourse of aphasic adults. *Clinical Aphasiology, 17,* 202-209.

Bradburn, N. (1969). *The structure of well-being.* Chicago: Aldine.

Brookshire, R. (1997). An introduction to neurogenic communication disorders, 5th edition. St. Louis: Mosby.

Chapey, R., Duchan, J., Elman, R., Garcia, L., Kagan, A., Lyon, J., & Simmons-Mackie, N. (2001). Life participation approach to aphasia: A statement of values for the future. In R. Chapey (Ed.). *Language intervention strategies in aphasia and related neurogenic communication disorders.* Philadelphia: Lippincott Williams & Wilkins, pp. 235-245.

Chapey, R., & Hallowell, B. (2001). Introduction to language intervention strategies in adult aphasia. In R. Chapey (Ed.), *Language intervention strategies in aphasia and related neurogenic communication disorders*. Philadelphia: Lippincott Williams & Wilkins, pp. 3-17.

Chubon, R. (1987). Development of a quality-of-life rating scale for use in health care evaluation. *Evaluation and the Health Professions, 10,* 186-200.

Davis, G.A., & Wilcox, M.J. (1985). *Adult aphasia rehabilitation: Applied pragmatics.* San Diego, CA: College-Hill Press.

DeShazer, S. (1997). Some thoughts on language use in therapy. *Contemporary Family Therapy, 19,* 133-141.

Elman, R., & Bernstein-Ellis, E. (1999). Aphasia group communication treatment: The Aphasia Center of California approach. In R. Elman (Ed.), *Group treatment of neurogenic communication disorders: The expert clinician's approach.* Boston, MA: Butterworth-Heinemann, pp. 47-56.

Kagan, A. (1998). Supported conversations for adults with aphasia: Methods and resources for training conversation partners. *Aphasiology, 12,* 816-830.

Kagan, A., Black, S., Duchan, J., Simmons-Mackie, N., & Square, P. (2001). Training volunteers as conversation partners using "Supported conversation for adults with Aphasia" (SCA): A controlled trial. *Journal of Speech, Language, and Hearing Research, 44,* 624-638.

Kagan, A., & Gailey, G. (1993). Functional is not enough: Training conversation partners for aphasic adults. In A. Holland & M. Forbes (Eds.), *Aphasia treatment: World perspectives.* San Diego, CA: Singular Publishing Group, pp. 199-215.

Kearns, K. (1989). Methodologies for studying generalization. In L.V. McReynolds & J. Spradlin (Eds.), *Generalization strategies in the treatment of communication disorders.* Toronto: BC Decker, pp. 13-30.

Larsen, R., Diener, R., & Emmons, R. (1985). An evaluation of subjective well-being measures. *Social Indicators Research, 17,* 1-17.

Lyon, J. (2000). Finding, defining, and refining functionality in real life for people confronting aphasia. In L. Worrall & C. Frattali (Eds.), *Neurogenic communication disorders: A functional approach.* New York: Thieme, pp.137-161.

Lyon, J., Cariski, D., Keisler, L., Rosenbek, J., Levine, R., Kumpula, J., Ryff, D., Coyne, S., & Levine, J. (1997). Communication partners: Enhancing participation in life and communication for adults with aphasia in natural settings. *Aphasiology, 11,* 693-708.

Lyon, J., & Shadden, B. (2001). Treating life consequences of aphasia's chronicity. In R. Chapey (Ed.), *Language intervention strategies in aphasia and related neurogenic communication disorders.* Philadelphia: Lippincott, Williams, & Wilkins, pp. 297-315.

National Stroke Association (2001). Uncontrollable stroke risk factors. *http://www.stroke.org/stroke_risk.cfm.*

Parr, S., Byng, S., & Gilpin, S. (1997). *Talking about aphasia: Living with loss of language after stroke.* Buckingham: Open University Press.

Pillari, V. (2002). *Social work practice: Theories and skills.* Boston: Allyn and Bacon.

Pound, C., Parr, S., & Duchan, J. (2001). Using partners' autobiographical reports to develop, deliver, and evaluate services in aphasia. *Aphasiology, 15,* 477-493.

Sacchett, C., Byng, S., Marshall, J., & Pound, C. (1999). Drawing together: Evaluation of a therapy programme for severe aphasia. *International Journal of Language and Communication Disorders, 34*, 265-289.

Simmons, N. (1993). *An ethnographic investigation of compensatory strategies in aphasia.* University Microfilms International: Ann Arbor, Michigan.

Simmons-Mackie, N., (2000). Social approaches to the management of aphasia. In L. Worrall & C. Frattali (Eds.), *Neurogenic communication disorders: A functional approach.* New York: Thieme, pp. 162-188.

Simmons-Mackie, N., & Damico, J. (1996). Accounting for handicaps in aphasia: Communicative assessment from an authentic social perspective. *Disability and Rehabilitation, 18*, 540-549.

Simmons-Mackie, N., & Damico, J. (1997). Reformulating the definition of compensatory strategies in aphasia. *Aphasiology, 8*, 761-781.

Simmons-Mackie, N., & Damico, J. (2001). Intervention outcomes: A clinical application of qualitative methods. *Topics in Language Disorders, 21*, 21-36.

Van Wormer, K. (1997). *Alcoholism Treatment: A social work perspective.* Chicago: Nelson Hall Publishing.

Vickers, C. (2003). Doing more with less for people with aphasia: Creative responses to healthcare change. *Speech Pathology Online, 1*, 1-7.

Wertz, R.T., Weiss, D., Aten, J., Brookshire, R., Garcia-Bunuel, L., Holland, A., Kurtzke, J., LaPointe, L., Milianti, F., Brannegan, R., Greenbaum, H., Marshall, R., Vogel, D., Carter, J., Barnes, N., & Goodman, R. (1986). Comparison of clinic, home, and deferred language treatment for aphasia: A Veterans Administration co-operative study. *Archives of Neurology, 43*, 576-586.

World Health Organization. (1980). *International classification if impairments, disabilities, and handicaps.* Geneva, Switzerland: WHO.

Worrall, L. (2000). A conceptual framework for a functional approach to acquired neurogenic disorders of communication and swallowing. In L. Worrall & C. Frattali (Eds.), *Neurogenic communication disorders: A functional approach.* New York: Thieme, pp. 3-18.

Worrall, L., & Yiu, E. (2000). Effectiveness of functional communication therapy by volunteers for people with aphasia following stroke. *Aphasiology, 14*, 911-924.

An Exploratory Study on Attitudes Toward Persons with Disabilities Among U.S. and Japanese Social Work Students

Reiko Hayashi
Mariko Kimura

SUMMARY. This exploratory study was conducted to understand and compare attitudes among social work students in the United States and Japan toward people with disabilities. The Modified Issues in Disabilities Scale (MIDS), designed to measure attitudes toward people with physical disabilities, was implemented on convenient samples of 92 U.S. and 73 Japanese social work students. The findings suggest that social work students in both countries hold moderately positive attitudes. Other similarities as well as differences among the sampled students from the two countries, and their implications to social work education, will be discussed in this paper. *[Article copies available for a fee from The Haworth Document Delivery Service: 1-800-HAWORTH. E-mail address: <docdelivery@ haworthpress.com> Website: <http://www.HaworthPress.com> © 2003 by The Haworth Press, Inc. All rights reserved.]*

Reiko Hayashi is Assistant Professor, School of Social Work, University of Utah, 395 S 1500 E, Salt Lake City, UT 84112.

Mariko Kimura is Professor, Social Work Department, Kwansei Gakuin University, 1-1-155 Uegahara, Nishinomiya, Hyogo 662-8501, Japan.

[Haworth co-indexing entry note]: "An Exploratory Study on Attitudes Toward Persons with Disabilities Among U.S. and Japanese Social Work Students." Hayashi, Reiko, and Mariko Kimura. Co-published simultaneously in *Journal of Social Work in Disability & Rehabilitation* (The Haworth Press, Inc.) Vol. 2, No. 2/3, 2003, pp. 65-85; and: *International Perspectives on Disability Services: The Same But Different* (ed: Francis K. O. Yuen) The Haworth Press, Inc., 2003, pp. 65-85. Single or multiple copies of this article are available for a fee from The Haworth Document Delivery Service [1-800-HAWORTH, 9:00 a.m. - 5:00 p.m. (EST). E-mail address: docdelivery@haworthpress.com].

10.1300/J198v02n02_05

KEYWORDS. Disability rights, disability paradigm, MIDS, attitude, social work students, Japan

Since the end of the World War II, there have been various levels of interactions between the United States and Japan: commercial, governmental, cultural, as well as grass roots. Both countries experienced the emergence of powerful disability rights movements in the 1960s and 1970s that were born alongside the other social movements of the time, among them the civil rights, anti-Vietnam war, students, environmental, and feminist movements (Hayashi & Okuhira, 2001). Disability rights organizations in both countries are among those groups that have maintained international exchanges over the last three decades. In the United States, this particular movement gave birth to the academic discipline of disability studies where the disability paradigm, a new way of understanding disability, has been explored (Pfeiffer, 1993). The disability paradigm, in turn, affected enactment of disability-related public policies (Silverstein, 2000).

Social work education in both countries, however, is slow to incorporate the issues of disability rights and the disability paradigm into their curricula. Given that social work education is not providing students proper information and skills regarding disability issues, this study explores students' attitudes toward people with disabilities. Current social work students in both countries will, as future practitioners, influence the lives of clients with disabilities. Understanding their attitudes will contribute to improving social work education and services in both countries.

These two countries that have had numerous exchanges also have differences in culture, disability-related policies, and histories of social work education. This paper will first describe the disability rights movement and the disability paradigm, their implications to social work education, and the interactions between the two countries in those areas. Then, it will present an exploratory study that utilizes the Modified Issues in Disabilities Scale (MIDS), a measure of attitudes toward persons with physical disabilities (Makas, 1993). The MIDS was formulated based on the concepts of the disability paradigm. This study seeks to understand and compare attitudes among social work students toward people with disabilities in the United States and in Japan. It will provide basic information to improve social work education and knowledge that will point the way to future research.

THE DISABILITY RIGHTS MOVEMENT
IN THE UNITED STATES

The medical model of disability, which has long enjoyed its status as the major perspective on disability in the United States, treats disability as a personal tragedy, something that should be "fixed" by professional intervention. In this view, those who cannot be cured are considered permanently deficient (Gilson & Depoy, 2000; Hahn, 1988; Mackelprang & Salsgiver, 1998).

The modern disability rights movement started in California in the 1960s and challenged the medical model. Ed Roberts, a quadriplegic and respirator user, entered the University of California-Berkeley in 1962, notwithstanding the reluctance of university officials and a complete lack of accommodations. Encouraged by his action, a dozen other students with severe disabilities enrolled at the university within the next few years. They formed a group known as the Rolling Quads and worked to make the campus and surrounding community accessible. Roberts also founded the first center for independent living in 1972 (Pelka, 1997, pp. 266-267; Shapiro, 1993, pp. 41-73). In New York, Judy Heumann, who won a disability-based discrimination lawsuit, became the first wheelchair-using teacher in New York City's public school system in 1970. She founded Disabled In Action, a political action group, and organized demonstrations and sit-ins protesting President Richard Nixon's veto of the Rehabilitation Act of 1972. She joined Roberts at the center for independent living in Berkeley in 1973. In 1977, disability rights activists occupied the federal building in San Francisco for 25 days, demanding the Carter administration implement Section 504 of the Rehabilitation Act of 1973. The action nurtured a sense of pride and solidarity in the disability community (Pelka, 1997, pp. 152-154; Shapiro, 1993, pp. 55-73). As the movement broadened its purview, disability rights advocates challenged the medical model that justified segregation and discrimination. Currently there are about 400 centers for independent living in the U.S. that are managed by disabled people and provide advocacy work as well as social services to support disabled people living in the community (DeJong, Batavia, & McKnew, 1992; Levy, 1988; Lifchez, 1979).

The academic discipline of disability studies emerged from the movement, and scholars have since been discussing the disability paradigm, a new way of understanding disability. The social constructionist model, a version of the disability paradigm, was well developed in the United States by the mid 1980s. This model emphasizes that environmental factors, not individual disabilities, play an important role in constructing the disability identity and that disabling environments are the source of problems, not the disabilities themselves. Since then, scholars and advocates have been introducing and discussing other versions such as the oppressed minority model, the independent living model, and the discrimination model. These versions may differ from one another in some ways, but they share a number of ideas: that disability is not a tragedy; does not mean dependency; does not mean a loss of potential, productivity, or social contribution; and is a natural part of the human experience. The disability paradigm also implies that professionals should not be the decision makers about the life of a person with a disability. While the medical model focuses on functional limitations of disabled individuals, the disability paradigm focuses on the whole person functioning in his or her environment (Pfeiffer, 1993). Since the 1970s, the disability paradigm has influenced the development of public policies and was articulated in the Americans With Disabilities Act (ADA) of 1990. The law identified disability issues as civil rights issues, and people with disabilities as oppressed members of society who deserve justice (Burgdorf, 1991; Silverstein, 2000; West, 1991). Some scholars of disability studies are also discussing a cultural model of disability that recognizes the shared identity of persons with disabilities and their community (Longmore, 1995).

SOCIAL WORK EDUCATION IN THE UNITED STATES

Professional social work has a long history in the United States, beginning with the friendly visitors of Charity Organization Societies and the settlement house movement in the 19th century. Professional social work education was established by the early 20th century (Abramovitz, 1988; Jansson, 1992), but the recognition of disability rights issues remained wanting until the enactment of the ADA (Quinn, 1995). In 1993, the Council on Social Work Education (CSWE) established the Ad Hoc Task Force on Social Work Education and Disability to study the issue. In 1997 the CSWE Board of Directors granted commission status to the task force, and 10 members were appointed to the new Commission on Disability and Persons with Disabilities (CDPD). The commission works to advance the inclusion of persons with disabilities as well as disability issues in social work education (Council on Social Work Education, 2003). An accommodation phrase for students with disabilities has been added to many social work syllabi as well as syllabi in other disciplines. Some schools now include disability issues in their curricula (Gilson, 2002). Further, job seekers in social work education may read in vacancy announcements a statement such as "women, people of color, and persons with disabilities are encouraged to apply." Awareness about disability rights among social workers and social work educators, however, is still wanting, and the medical model still holds sway in the social work practice field (Hiranandani, in press).

THE DISABILITY RIGHTS MOVEMENT IN JAPAN

A disability rights movement in Japan was also born in 1960s-1970s. At that time the moral model of disabilities (Mackelprang & Salsgiver, 1998) was entrenched in Japanese society. Disabilities were seen as punishment, and those with disabilities were looked down upon. It was assumed that they were suffering the consequence of transgressions they or their parents made in their current or previous lives. The medical model of disabilities was also pervasive then, emphasizing cure as the foremost life goal for people with disabilities (Longmore, 1985; Mackelprang & Salsgiver, 1998). As a result of these cultural views, many disabled people led lives segregated from the nondisabled society in their secluded pursuits of cures. In response to this social situation, where people with disabilities and their families were stigmatized and forced to live in shame, disability activists took direct action. They organized protests against human rights violations in residential institutions; criticized discriminatory societal policies and practices, and demanded integrated schools, access to transportation, and support for community living. In the process, they helped raise the awareness of both the disabled and the wider Japanese society about the need for civil rights for people with disabilities (Hayashi & Okuhira, 2001).

One of the issues that disability advocates opposed strongly was the call for a "Compulsory K-12 Special Education System." Unfortunately, the national government implemented the system in 1979, creating separate special education schools for children with disabilities. Elementary, junior high, and high schools for special education were established as well as the Visiting Teacher Programs that send teachers to the homes of disabled children to provide educational instruction. While implementation of these systems did reduce the number of disabled children exempted from primary education (Ministry of Education, Culture, Sports, Science, and Technology [MECSST], 2002), it also institutionalized the segregation of children with disabilities from the larger society.

An important pertinent event of the following decade was the 1981 International Year of Disabled Persons, which prompted advocates from the United States to visit Japan. Ed Roberts and Judy Heumann, described in the U.S. section above, were among those visitors. These U.S. advocates introduced to Japan the concept of independent living centers. Run by people with disabilities, these centers were providing advocacy work and services for disabled persons living in American communities (DeJong et al., 1992; Lifchez, 1979). The advocates invited some Japanese persons with disabilities to be trained in the U.S. to manage such facilities. The first independent living center in Japan was established in 1986 and staffed mainly by those trained in the United States (Hayashi & Okuhira, 2001). Also during the 1980s, disability rights organizations in Japan shifted their focus from leading protests in response to discriminatory incidents to proactively negotiating with regional governments to improve the daily lives of disabled persons. As a result of these efforts, the first publicly funded personal attendants program for disabled persons living in the community was started in Osaka City in 1986 (Onoue, 2000).

By 2000, there were 90 independent living centers in Japan. They provide services to people with disabilities living in the community as well as negotiate with governmental agencies to increase official support for attendant services (JIL, 2000). The national and regional governments have come to accept that segregation cannot provide the best quality of life for disabled persons and that organizations run by disabled persons can be competent service providers. The Government Action Plan for Persons With Disabilities of 1995 shows a change in governmental policies toward the promotion of disabled persons living in the community (Ministry of Health, Labor, and Welfare [MHLW], 2002a).

In academia, the Japan Society for Disability Studies was established in 1999. Although still small in numbers, active scholars of disability studies work with the disability rights organizations and cooperate with scholars in the Unites States (Kuramoto & Nagase, 2000).

SOCIAL WORK EDUCATION IN JAPAN

In Japan, social welfare issues had been mainly handled by local government agencies whose employees rarely had training in the social welfare field or held social work degrees. In 1987, however, the Social Worker and Care Worker Act was enacted and established the professional status of people working in the social welfare field. National exams for social work and psychiatric social work certifications were implemented for eligible applicants (MHLW, 2002b). The Japanese Association of Certified Social Workers (JACSW, 2002), Japan's counterpart of the National Association of Social Workers in the United States, was founded in 1993. The Long-Term Care Insurance Act of 1997 further expanded opportunities for social work professionals. Several levels of additional professional and paraprofessional certifications for those who work in the long-term care system were created in addition to "social workers" and "psychiatric social workers." In response to these demands, many social work programs were created in four-year universities, junior colleges, and technical schools. Depending on their educational levels, graduates of those programs could apply for various levels of national certification exams (MHLW, 2002b). The professionalization of social work in Japan is now a reality.

While the social work educational system has developed rapidly in the last 10 years, disability rights issues have not yet been required in its curricula. It remains up to individual educators to include the perspectives of people with disabilities. The inclusion of disability issues in curricula may increase in Japan since their schools of social work are expanding interactions with social work educators in the United States, where the inclusion is strongly encouraged.

RATIONALE AND RESEARCH QUESTIONS

The two countries have had numerous exchanges, especially in the second half of the 20th century. Disability rights advocates in both countries have also influenced the development of public policies that have improved the lives of people with disabilities. Social work education in both countries, however, has been slow to incorporate the issues of disability rights in the curricula. It is the authors' interest as social work educators, one in Japan and the other in the United States, to explore and compare social work students' attitudes toward people with disabilities. Today's social work students in both countries will, as future practitioners, influence the lives of clients with disabilities. Social workers with positive attitudes toward disability rights and people with disabilities can play an advocacy role as allies for clients with disabilities. On the other hand, social workers with prejudice against people with disabilities can disempower their clients.

In the United States, lawsuits have been filed under the ADA, some of which have been reported in the media (Pardeck, 1999). As a result, U.S. social work students may be more aware of disability rights issues even though their schools may not yet offer courses on disabilities. Although Japan has no law equivalent to the ADA, the social norms may have changed there as well through the global exchange of ideas since the 1981 International Year of Disabled Persons and through the advocacy work done by independent living centers and other groups. With government policies now promoting more inclusion of people with disabilities in community living (MHLW, 2002a), today's Japanese students may be more accepting of people with disabilities than in previous generations. On the other hand, because of the Japan's segregated K-12 school system, Japanese students who have little contact with disabled persons may be as prejudiced as ever.

Although the authors would like to study relationships between the students' attitudes and social work education, changes in societal norms, disability-related policies, and international exchanges between the two countries, they leave the extensive research for the future. As a first step, this study examines social work students' attitude toward disabled persons, and the similarity and differences in attitudes among U.S. and Japanese students. This paper provides information about the disability rights movements, disability-related policies, social work education, and the history of international exchange as background knowledge to ponder.

Specific research questions for this study were:

1. Do Japanese and U.S. social work students overall have positive or negative attitudes toward persons with physical disabilities?
2. Do Japanese and U.S. social work students have different attitudes in specific areas such as education, law, and physiological and psychological characteristics of disabled persons?
3. Does educational level play a role in their attitudes?
4. Do opportunities to have contacts with persons with disabilities affect their attitudes?

RESEARCH METHODS

Samples

Convenient samples of 48 undergraduate and 44 graduate social work students attending a university on the west coast of the United States and 38 undergraduate and 35 "professional school" social work students in Japan participated in the study. All of the students sampled were taking a course from one of the authors. U.S. and Japanese undergraduate students were primarily juniors and seniors. In Japan there is no program equivalent to the MSW programs in the U.S. Consequently, the authors chose students from a "professional social work school." These schools were established to train people who have undergraduate degrees in areas other than social work. The students can obtain a social work diploma in two years, while a regular undergraduate social work degree requires four years of schooling. They are nontraditional students who have some work experience in the social welfare field. The authors considered these students similar to U.S. graduate students, at least in terms of age and experience in the field of social work.

Instrument

The Modified Issues in Disabilities Scale (MIDS; Makas, 1993) was administered to the participants during one of their regularly scheduled classes. The MIDS was created based on the disability paradigm that values civil rights and independence of people with disabilities. The scale was translated into Japanese for the Japanese students.

The instrument gathers demographic information from participants: gender, age, race/ethnicity, presence or absence of disability, and amount of contact with persons with disabilities. A "contact" variable had five value levels: no contact, very little contact, some contact, quite a bit of contact, and a great deal of contact.

The MIDS is a 33-item self-report Likert-scale questionnaire intended to measure both cognitive and affective components of attitudes toward persons with physical disabilities. Participants are asked to indicate the degree to which they agree with a particular statement, with responses ranging from 1 (strongly disagree) to 7 (strongly agree), with 4 (the midpoint) representing no opinion. To minimize the possibilities of response set bias, 15 statements were written so that "strongly agree" (7) indicated the most positive attitude toward people with disabilities, while the remaining 18 statements were written so that "strongly disagree" (1) indicated the most positive attitude. For analysis, the latter 18 were reverse-scored so higher scores would indicate more positive attitudes.

The scale includes statements about people with physical disabilities in general as well as statements about three specific disability groups: blindness/visual impairment (a visible, sensory disability); mobility impairment (a visible, nonsensory disability); and hidden disabilities, including diabetes, cancer, and epilepsy (invisible, nonsensory disabilities). The scale measures participants' attitudes in several areas, including education (e.g., "The majority of adolescents with physical disabilities should attend special schools which are specifically designed to meet their needs"), laws (e.g., "Zoning laws should not prohibit group homes for people with disabilities from being established in residential districts"), contact with disabled persons (e.g., "If you are talking to a blind person, it is all right to use words such as 'see' or 'look' in a conversation"), physiological abilities of disabled persons (e.g., "Drivers with physical disabilities have more automobile accidents than drivers without disabilities"), and psychological characteristics of disabled persons (e.g.,"People who have disabilities are generally no more anxious or tense than people who do not have disabilities" (Makas, Finnerty-Fried, Sigafoos, & Reiss, 1988).

DATA ANALYSIS AND FINDINGS

Two questionnaires that had more than three blanks were considered invalid and eliminated. The final data included 163 participants. Blanks up to the maximum of three were coded as "4" (Makas, 1993). The 18 reverse-scored statements created to minimize the response set bias were recoded with higher scores indicating more positive attitudes.

The scores of the 33 statements were added and the variable MIDS Total was created. The higher the MIDS Total score, the more positive a participant's attitude is toward persons with physical disabilities. The possible range of "MIDS Total" was 231 (the highest score) to 33 (the lowest score).

Demographics

Table 1 shows the demographic information of participants. More than 83% of the participants were female. The mean ages of the participants were 23.2 and 27.6 in undergraduate samples in Japan and the U.S. respectively, 31.4 for the Japanese professional school students, and 32.1 for the graduate students in the U.S. Only one Japanese student out of 73 (1.4%) had a disability while 12 out of 90 (13.3%) U.S. students were disabled.

The authors asked participants about the amount of contact they had had with persons with disabilities. The five value levels were no contact, very little contact, some contact, quite a bit of contact, and a great deal of contact. Table 2 shows the findings. While more than 40% of respondents had no or very little contact with persons with disabilities, and 29% responded to have had quite a bit of or a great deal of contact with persons with disabilities.

TABLE 1. Demographics

Groups	Number of participants	Mean age	Students with disabilities	Gender Female	Male
Japan undergraduate	38	23.2 (sd = 7.2)	0 (0%)	38 (100%)	0 (0%)
Japan professional school	35	31.4 (sd = 9.8)	1 (2.9%)	22 (63%)	13 (37%)
U.S. undergraduate	48	27.6 (sd = 8.5)	8 (16.7%)	40 (83%)	8 (17%)
U.S. graduate	42	32.1 (sd = 7.4)	4 (9.5%)	36 (86%)	6 (14%)

TABLE 2. Contact with Persons with Disabilities

Groups	No contact	Very little contact	Some contact	Quite a bit of contact	A great deal of contact	Number of participants
Japan undergraduate	14 (36.8%)	12 (31.6%)	4 (10.5%)	3 (7.9%)	5 (13.2%)	38 (100%)
Japan professional school	3 (9.1%)	9 (27.3%)	8 (24.2%)	7 (21.2%)	6 (18.2%)	33 (100%)
U.S. undergraduate	2 (4.3%)	10 (21.3%)	17 (36.2%)	9 (19.1%)	9 (19.1%)	47 (100%)
U.S. graduate	2 (5.0%)	14 (35.0%)	18 (45.0%)	2 (5.0%)	4 (10.0%)	40 (100%)
Total	21 (13.3%)	45 (28.5%)	47 (29.7%)	21 (13.3%)	24 (15.2%)	158 (100%)

All participants in Japan were racially and ethnically Japanese. Table 3 shows the diverse racial and ethnic backgrounds of the U.S. students. The U.S. university is located in a city on the west coast populated by many racial and ethnic groups. The student body also includes many first-generation immigrants from Asian countries and Latin America, as well as other international students. Therefore, the U.S. samples include both immigrants and international students. Since the authors did not ask their nations of origin in the survey, they do not have the ratio of foreign-born students in the data.

The MIDS Total Score

The Cronbach alpha coefficient for the MIDS scale was 0.77 for this study. The mean MIDS total score was 157.85 (sd = 17.9), with a range of 104-211. Dividing 157.85 by the number of statements (33) gives a

TABLE 3. Race/Ethnicity of the U.S. Students

Race/Ethnicity	Number
African American/Black	6
Asian/Pacific Islander	24
Latino	16
Caucasian	21
Biracial/Mixed	13
(Missing)	10
Total	90

mean statement score of 4.78, which shows an overall moderately positive response. To check the tendency to choose positive or negative responses to the statements, the authors counted the number of positive responses (values 5, 6, and 7) and negative responses (values 1, 2, and 3) for each participant. The result showed that 149 (91.4%) participants chose more positive responses than negative ones. Table 4 presents the minimum, maximum, and mean MIDS total scores for each group.

T-Tests and Correlation

Table 5 presents gender differences in MIDS total scores in both countries. T-tests showed no significant gender difference in MIDS total scores among Japanese students ($t = -.376$ $df = 71$ $p = .71$) and a significant gender difference among U.S. students ($t = -2.139$ $df = 88$ $p = .035$). U.S. females had significantly more positive attitudes than U.S. males.

There was also a small but a significant correlation between "contact" and MIDS total score (Pearson $r = .22, p < .01$), demonstrating that the more contact one has, the better the attitudes toward persons with disabilities.

Analysis of Variance

Data were screened to ensure that the assumptions of Analysis of Variance were fulfilled. One outlier was altered to a value that is within the extreme tail in the accepted distribution. Then, the authors conducted a one-way analysis of variance to examine the differences in attitudes among the four samples. The independent variable was group affiliation; the dependent variable was the MIDS total. The result, presented in Table 6, shows a significant difference in MIDS total scores

TABLE 4. MIDS Total Scores[a] Based on Country and Education Level

Groups	N	Min	Max	Mean	sd
Japan undergraduate	38	126	176	152.00	12.42
Japan professional school	35	129	202	157.71	15.06
U.S. undergraduate	48	104	188	152.35	17.99
U.S. graduate	42	137	211	169.52	18.98
Total	163	104	211	157.85	17.89

[a]*Note.* The possible range of "MIDS Total" is 231 (the highest score) to 33 (the lowest score).

TABLE 5. MIDS Total Scores[a] Based on Country and Gender

Gender	N	Min	Max	Mean	sd
Japan male	13	129	177	153.31	13.83
Japan female	60	126	202	155.05	14.07
U.S. male	14	104	183	149.93	18.81
U.S. female	76	121	211	102.29	20.05

TABLE 6. Analysis of Variance

	SS	df	MS	F	p
Between groups	8480.194	3	2826.731	10.575	.000
Within groups	42501.855	159	267.307		
Total	50982.049	162			

among the four groups ($F(3,159) = 10.58$, $p < .0005$). The Scheffe's post hoc test revealed that U.S. graduate students scored significantly higher than the other three groups. There were no statistical significant differences among the other three groups.

Item Analyses

Values of 1 and 2 ("very negative attitudes") and 6 and 7 ("very positive attitudes") were counted for each statement for each group. Figures 1a, 1b, 2a, 2b, and 2c show the results of selected statements.

The statement that received the most "very negative attitudes" by all groups was, "Most people who have physical disabilities expect no more love and reassurance than anyone else." More than 71% of the

Group 1 Figures Responses Showing "Very Negative Attitudes" on Selected Statements

FIGURE 1a. Disagree or Strongly Disagree with Statement: "Most People Who Have Physical Disabilities Expect No More Love and Reassurance Than Anyone Else."

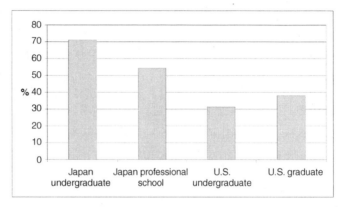

FIGURE 1b. Agree or Strongly Agree with Statement: "For a Person with a Severe Disability, the Kindness of Others Is More Important Than Any Educational Program."

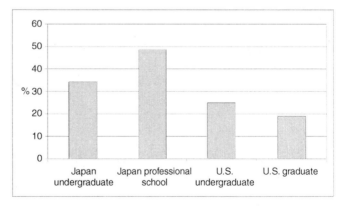

Japanese undergraduate and 54% of the professional school students disagreed or strongly disagreed with the statement, as did more than 31% of the U.S. undergraduate and 38% graduate students. No Japanese undergraduate students, and only 3 (8.6%) Japanese professional school students, agreed or strongly agreed with the statement. In contrast,

Group 2 Figures Responses Showing "Very Positive Attitudes" on Selected Statements

FIGURE 2a. Disagree or Strongly Disagree with Statement: "People with Physical Disabilities Should Get Special Certification from Their Physicians in Order to Apply for a Marriage License."

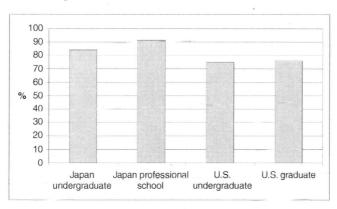

FIGURE 2b. Agree or Strongly Agree with Statement: "Zoning Laws Should Not Prohibit Group Homes for People with Disabilities from Being Established in Residential Districts."

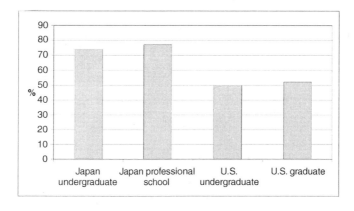

FIGURE 2c. Agree or Strongly Agree with Statement: "It Is Logical for a Woman Who Uses a Wheelchair to Consider Having a Baby."

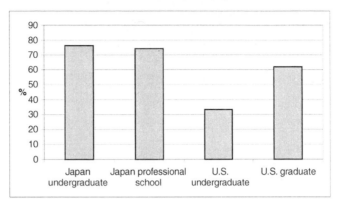

nearly 40% of U.S. undergraduate and 48% graduate students agreed or strongly agreed with the statement, exceeding their percentages for "very negative attitudes." The responses of Japanese students for this statement skewed to "very negative attitudes," while the responses of U.S. students were spread more evenly from positive to negative.

The statement that received the second most "very negative attitudes" by Japanese students was "For a person with a severe disability, the kindness of others is more important than any educational program." More than 34% of undergraduate and 48% of professional school students agreed or strongly agreed with the statement, while only 18% of undergraduate and 5.8% of professional school students disagreed or strongly disagreed. In contrast, 48% of U.S. graduate students disagreed or strongly disagreed with the statement, while only 19% of them agreed or strongly agreed. As for U.S. undergraduates, 25% agreed and 21% disagreed. Japanese students are more likely than U.S. students to believe that persons with physical disabilities are more in need of affection than nondisabled persons and that the kindness of others is more important to them than education.

On the positive side, Japanese undergraduates (84.2%), Japanese professional students (91.4%), and U.S. undergraduates (75.0%) disagreed or strongly disagreed with the statement "People with physical disabilities should get special certification from their physicians in order to apply for a marriage license." This statement received the most "very positive attitudes" among those three groups. More than 76% of

U.S. graduate students also disagreed or strongly disagreed with the statement. It was their fifth most positive response. No Japanese students agreed or strongly agreed with the statement, while 3 (6.3%) U. S. undergraduate and 4 (9.5%) graduate students did. The statement "It is more humane to allow a child with a severe disability to die at birth than for her/him to live as a person with a severe disability" received the most "disagree" and "strongly disagree" responses from U.S. graduate students (85.7%). The majority of Japanese undergraduate (68.4%), professional students (68.6%), and U.S. undergraduates (64.6%) also disagreed with the statement.

The statement "It is logical for a woman who uses a wheelchair to consider having a baby" also received high positive responses from Japanese students. Seventy-six percent of Japanese undergraduates and 74% of professional students agreed or strongly agreed with the statement, while only 33% of U.S. undergraduates and 62% of graduate students agreed or strongly agreed with the statement. This finding of a high percentage of Japanese students accepting the marriage and parenthood of persons with disabilities shows a change in the social norm in a positive direction over time. In the 1960s and 1970s, Japanese society did not consider the possibility of marriage and parenthood for people with disabilities. Women with disabilities at that time were often coerced into having hysterectomies (Hayashi & Okuhira, 2001).

The statement "Zoning laws should not prohibit group homes for people with disabilities from being established in residential districts" received high positive responses from Japanese students as well. While 74% of Japanese undergraduates and 77% of professional school students agreed or strongly agreed with the statement, only 50% of U.S. undergraduates and 52% of graduate students agreed or strongly agreed.

All statements that related to civil rights received high rankings in positive responses. It appears that the majority of participants believed that persons with disabilities should be treated equally with nondisabled citizens under the law in terms of marriage license, automobile insurance, income tax, zoning laws, the right to procreate, and the right to live.

DISCUSSION

Only 1 Japanese student out of 73 had a disability, while 10 out of 69 U.S. students were disabled. This may be a result of segregated Japanese K-12 school systems where students with disabilities in the special education schools are not encouraged to go on to college. Further, there is no law in Japan to require institutions of higher education to support students with disabilities. In contrast, U.S. universities usually have offices that provide services to students with disabilities. Perhaps Japanese students with disabilities have hesitated to "come out" even in the anonymous survey because they were afraid of being labeled, while U.S. students felt less stigmatized. In any case, it is important that the Japanese social work education system support the pursuit of social work careers by students with disabilities. The long-term care field is an important and fast-growing area. The voices of social workers with disabilities who can bring their own experiences to the field will be a great asset to the service system in Japan.

Students of both countries showed moderately positive attitudes overall toward people with disabilities. The moral model of disabilities that was prevalent in Japan decades ago seems to have subsided, at least among this sample of social work students. The medical model that emphasizes that disabled persons must be cured to be accepted by society also failed to be a leading perspective in those samples. Although the scale does not include items directly discussing a cure, participants of both countries appeared to accept disabled persons as they are. Even though Japan does not have a civil rights law for people with disabilities, Japanese participants tended to agree with statements that support equal treatment for disabled and nondisabled citizens. It is encouraging that students from both countries responded positively regarding the civil rights of people with disabilities.

Although the findings show a tendency of participants to accept disabled persons in terms of their rights, they also reveal negative opinions in the area of "psychological characteristics of disabled persons." Many participants, especially Japanese students, believed that disabled persons need more love and assurance than nondisabled persons, and that the kindness of others is more important than education for disabled persons. This may come from the fact that people with disabilities are not yet integrated into the Japanese society, and participants tend to assume that people with disabilities are more needy and weaker beings.

A t-test showed that there is a significant gender difference in attitudes among U.S. students but not among Japanese students. This result concurs with previous research on U.S. college students that females tend to have more positive attitudes than males toward people with disabilities (Esses & Beaufoy, 1994; Granello & Wheaton, 2001).

Another difference between the two countries is that Japanese students tend to have smaller standard deviations in MIDS total scores than U.S. students. This may stem from a more homogeneous culture that encourages more homogeneous opinions in Japan.

A Pearson correlation analysis showed the small but significant result that the more contact people have, the better their attitudes toward persons with disabilities become. This indicates the necessity for schools of social work in both countries to recruit and support students and faculty with disabilities. The presence of more people with disabilities in the educational system would improve overall attitudes.

Analysis of Variance shows that U.S. graduate students scored significantly higher than the other three groups. They may be more aware of the disability rights issues through their longer experiences in the social work field and the graduate courses.

A limitation of this research is that it focuses only on attitudes toward people with physical disabilities. As social work professionals also work with people with disabilities other than physical (psychiatric, intellectual, and learning disabilities) and with multiple disabilities, further research will be necessary to evaluate the attitudes of social work students toward people with these other conditions.

Another limitation is that the findings cannot be generalized beyond the samples. They were convenient samples that are not necessarily representative of social work students in both countries. The U.S. samples were taken from a school that is located in an ethnically and racially diverse area of the United States. Different demographic configurations may produce different responses to the scale. Further and more rigorous study is necessary to gain a more well defined understanding of the attitudes toward people with disabilities among social work students in both countries.

In conclusion, it is encouraging that the social work students in this study did not show overall negative attitudes. The average score for all students was 4.78, which is just above a 4, meaning "Don't know/No opinion," and considerably below a 7, which is the most desirable attitude in the Likert Scale. So there is much room for improvement. The accomplishments by the disability rights movements and disability studies in the last three decades need to be incorporated into social work education in both countries. The curricula of schools of social work should provide more disability content that promotes the civil rights of people with disabilities, leads to the eradication of prejudices against disabled people, and encourages disability pride among students with disabilities.

REFERENCES

Abramovitz, M. (1988). *Regulating the lives of women: Social welfare policy from colonial times to the present.* Boston, MA: South End Press.

Americans With Disabilities Act (ADA). (1990). PL 101-336, 42 U.S.C. Section 12101.

Burgdorf, R. (1991). The Americans with Disabilities Act: Analysis and implications of a second-generation civil rights statute. *Harvard Civil Rights/Civil Liberties Law Review, 26,* 413-522.

Council on Social Work Education (CSWE). (2002). Commission on disability and persons with disabilities. Retrieved February 3, 2003 from http://www.cswe.org/.

DeJong, G., Batavia, A., & McKnew, L. (1992). The independent living model of personal assistance in long-term-care policy. *Generations, 16,* 89-95.

Esses, V., & Beaufoy, S. (1994). Determinants of attitudes toward people with disabilities. *Journal of Social Behavior and Personality, 9*(5), 43-64.

Gilson, S. F. (Ed.). (2002). *Integrating disability content in social work education.* Alexandria, VA: Council on Social Work Education.

Gilson, S. F., & Depoy, E. (2000). Multiculturalism and disability: A critical perspective. *Disability & Society, 15*(2), 207-218.

Granello, D., & Wheaton, J. (2001). Attitudes of undergraduate students toward persons with physical disabilities and mental illness. *Journal of Applied Rehabilitation Counseling, 32*(3), 9-16.

Hahn, H. (1988). The politics of physical differences: Disability and discrimination. *Journal of Social Issues, 44,* 39-47.

Hayashi, R., & Okuhira, M. (2001). The disability rights movement in Japan: Past, present, and future. *Disability & Society, 16*(6), 855-869.

Hiranandani, V. S. (in press). Rethinking disability in social work: Interdisciplinary perspectives. In G. May, M. Raske, & C. Baker (Eds.), *Disability and social work.* Boston, MA: Allyn and Bacon.

Jansson, B. (1992). *The reluctant welfare state: American social welfare policies.* Belmont, CA: Wadsworth.

Japan Council on Independent Living Centers (JIL). (2002). *Japan Council on Independent Living Centers.* Retrieved February 3, 2003 from *http://www.d1.dion.ne.jp/~jil.*

Japanese Association of Certified Social Workers (JACSW). (2002). *Japanese Association of Certified Social Workers.* Retrieved February 3, 2003 from *http://www. jacsw.or.jp/.*

Kuramoto, T., & Nagase, O. (2000). *Shougaigaku o kataru [Disability studies].* Tokyo, Japan: Empowerment Institute.

Levy, C. W. (1988). *A people's history of the independent living movement.* Lawrence: University of Kansas.

Lifchez, R. (1979). *Design for independent living.* Berkeley: University of California Press.

Longmore, P. K. (1995). The second phase: From disability rights to disability culture. *The Disability Rag and Resources, 16*(5), 4-11.

Longmore, P. K. (1985). Screening stereotypes: Images of disabled people. *Social Policy, 16,* 31-37.

Mackelprang, R. W., & Salsgiver, R. O. (1998). *Disability: A diversity model approach in human service practice.* Pacific Grove, CA: Brooks/Cole.

Makas, E. (1993). *The MIDS: Modified Issues in Disability Scale, Transitional Version.* Lewiston, ME: Lewiston-Auburn College of the University of Southern Maine.

Makas, E., Finnerty-Fried, P., Sigafoos, A., & Reiss, D. (1988). The issues in disability scale: A new cognitive & affective measure of attitudes toward people with physical disabilities. *Journal of Applied Rehabilitation Counseling, 19*(1), 21-29.

Ministry of Education, Culture, Sports, Science and Technology (MECSST). (2001). 21-seikino tokushukyoikuno arikatanituite [Special education in 21st century] Final report chapter 1, Tokyo, Japan: MECSST. Retrieved February 3, 2003 from *http://www.mext.go.jp/a_menu/shotou/shingi/shotou06.htm.*

Ministry of Health, Labor, and Welfare (MHLW). (2002a). Review of health and welfare measures for people with disabilities. *Annual report on health and welfare: 1998-1999 social security and national life.* Tokyo, Japan. Retrieved February 3, 2003 from *http://www1.mhlw.go.jp/english/wp_5/vol1/p2c4s2.html.*

Ministry of Health, Labor, and Welfare (MHLW). (2002b). Establishment of the long-term care insurance system and the development of long-term care service supply system. *Annual report on health and welfare: 1998-1999 social security and national life.* Tokyo, Japan. Retrieved February 3, 2003 from *http://www1.mhlw. go.jp/english/wp_5/vol1/p2c2s2.html.*

Onoue, K. (2000). Osaka-si zensin syogaisya kaigonin haken jigyo hassokuno keika [The process of establishing the home attendants program for disabled persons in Osaka City]. *SSK KHJ, 1517*, pp. 48-49.

Pardeck, J. T. (1999). Disability discrimination in social work education: Current issues for social work programs and faculty. *Journal of Teaching in Social Work, 19*(1/2), 151-163.

Pelka, F. (1997). *The disability rights movement.* Santa Barbara, CA: ABC-CLIO.

Pfeiffer, D. (1993). Overview of the disability movement: History, legislative record, and political implications. *Policy Studies Journal, 21*, 724-34.

Quinn, P. (1995). Social work education and disability: Benefiting from the impact of the ADA. *Journal of Teaching in Social Work, 12*(1/2), 55-71.

Shapiro, J. P. (1993). *No pity: People with disabilities forging a new civil rights movement.* New York: Times Books.

Silverstein, R. (2000). Federal disability policy framework. *The Iowa Law Review, 85*, 1691-1798.

West, J. (1991). *The Americans With Disabilities Act: From policy to practice.* New York: Milbank Memorial Fund.

Max versus *Max:*
Disability-Related Services
in the U.S. and Germany

Ute C. Orgassa

SUMMARY. Disability-related services and experiences of the United States of America and Germany are compared. A fictional case example concerning a person with a developmental disability is followed from birth to adulthood. Examples of possible life choices are given. *[Article copies available for a fee from The Haworth Document Delivery Service: 1-800-HAWORTH. E-mail address: <docdelivery@haworthpress.com> Website: <http://www.HaworthPress.com> © 2003 by The Haworth Press, Inc. All rights reserved.]*

KEYWORDS. Developmental disability, detection, intervention, disability-related services, USA and Germany

INTRODUCTION

In this article the author compares disability-related services between two countries, the U.S. and Germany. This is done by the use of a purely fictional case example. The case example itself is designed to be identical for both countries, so the disability of the child and the family situa-

---

Ute C. Orgassa resides in Pasadena, CA.

[Haworth co-indexing entry note]: "Max versus *Max:* Disability-Related Services in the U.S. and Germany." Orgassa, Ute C. Co-published simultaneously in *Journal of Social Work in Disability & Rehabilitation* (The Haworth Press, Inc.) Vol. 2, No. 2/3, 2003, pp. 87-100; and: *International Perspectives on Disability Services: The Same But Different* (ed: Francis K. O. Yuen) The Haworth Press, Inc., 2003, pp. 87-100. Single or multiple copies of this article are available for a fee from The Haworth Document Delivery Service [1-800-HAWORTH, 9:00 a.m. - 5:00 p.m. (EST). E-mail address: docdelivery@haworthpress.com].

10.1300/J198v02n02_06

tion regarding relatives are in both countries exactly the same. The life circumstances of those relatives and the service opportunities they encounter, however, are tailored to more typical situations in each respective country.

Caution

However, if the author compares services in the U.S. and Germany, they have to do this with certain cautions in mind. First, disability services in the U.S. differ considerably from state to state, and even within the states there are differences among school districts and in general between rural and urban service areas.

In Germany there are not as many differences in regard to mandated services, but there are considerable differences in availability of service providers and service options between the former Western (old) and former Eastern (new) states. So *where* the author locates the case example within the two countries makes a difference. Also other factors like knowing leaders in the community, being an outspoken versus a reclusive parent, or simply luck play defining roles in regard to experiences with the service system. Last, this example can only be a crude generalization regarding things that are more likely to happen than others. In the end, every disability experience is unique.

THE CASE EXAMPLE

Max is born with a congenital intellectual disability. He will be able to walk, get dressed by himself, talk in simple sentences, and do simple tasks after they have been explained and demonstrated to him. He will not be able to read and write besides some short words and phrases and his name. He will be required to wear glasses and orthopedic shoes. He will have a slight congenital heart defect that does not bother him much but needs to be monitored. He will not be able to follow lengthy conversations, think in the abstract, or understand the meaning of more complex concepts (like money). He will be able to know the difference between right and wrong, success and failure, and the value of friendship.

Max is born to a single working mother in her middle 20s. He has no siblings at the time. They live in an urban area, and the mother has a fairly functional support network. They live in California for the U.S. example and in Northrhein-Westfalia (NRW) for the Germany example.

Definition of Disability

Max would be defined as a person with a developmental disability in the U.S. and as a person with a cognitive disability in Germany. Simply the way those terms are used and defined can be confusing, because different laws define disability in different ways. In the United States there are several definitions of disabilities. Different legislation uses various definitions, and sometimes those definitions are broad in scope; some times contradict each other (Berkowitz, 1987); and sometimes they are specific only to the developmental disability. The current specific definition of developmental disability is in the Developmental Disabilities Assistance and Bill of Rights Act of 1990 (1990) and reads as follows:

> Developmental Disability means a severe, chronic disability of a person 5 years of age or older that (A) is attributable to a mental or physical impairment or combination of mental and physical impairments, (B) is manifested before the person attains age 22, (C) is likely to continue indefinitely, (D) results in substantial functional limitations in three or more of the following areas of major life activity: (i) self-care, (ii) receptive and expressive language, (iii) learning, (iv) mobility, (v) self-direction, (vi) capacity for independent living, and (viii) economic self-sufficiency, (E) reflects the person's need for a combination and sequence of special, interdisciplinary, or generic care, treatment, or other services which are of lifelong or extended duration and are individually planned and coordinated; except that such term, when applied to infants and young children means individuals from birth to age 5, inclusive, who have substantial developmental delay or specific congenital or acquired conditions with a high probability of resulting in developmental disabilities if services are not provided. (p. 1192)

This definition highlights the need of persons with developmental disabilities for services in the pursuit of an independent and self-directed life. It does not exclude persons with rare impairments like needs-based disabilities, which compile lists of eligible definitions. Max qualifies under this particular definition because he has limitations in several areas of major life activity, needs services, and his disability is detected before age 18. The current general definition of disability can be found in the Americans With Disabilities Act of 1990 (1990) and defines disability as: "(A) a physical or mental impairment that substantially limits one or more major life activities of such individual; (B) a record of such impairment; or (C) being regarded as having such an impairment" (p. 330).

Also, because Max is most likely to be defined as having mental retardation, the current American Association on Mental Retardation (AAMR) definition of mental retardation will be used and reads as follows:

> Mental retardation refers to substantial limitations in present functioning. It is characterized by significantly subaverage intellectual functioning, existing concurrently with related limitations in two or more of the following applicable adaptive skill areas: communication, self-care, home living, social skills, community use, self-direction, health and safety, functional academics, leisure, and work. Mental retardation manifests before age 18. (Luckasson, Coulter, Polloway, Reiss, Schalock, Snell, Spitalnik, & Stark, 1992, p. 1)

This definition includes systems of support on an individual basis; however, most professionals still work with the second-to-last definition of mental retardation that includes the mild, moderate, severe, and profound categories along IQ points. The latest definition that rejected those categories and uses systems of support instead is not yet widely utilized. Therefore, at this point in time in the U.S., Max would most likely be categorized as a child with moderate mental retardation.

In Germany there is not a clear-cut overall IQ distinction when it comes to disability definitions. The definitions used in the different laws and also in common use look more at the capabilities and no capabilities of the persons concerned. A general disability definition used in Germany is the one of the World Health Organization (WHO). WHO's International Classification of Impairments, Disability, and Handicap acknowledges the multiple facets of disability and defines impairment as:

> Any temporary or permanent loss or abnormality of a body structure or function, whether physiological or psychological. An impairment is a disturbance affecting functions that are essentially mental (memory, consciousness) or sensory, internal organs (heart, kidney), the head, the trunk, or the limbs. (Babotte, Grillemin, Nearkasen, & the Lorhandicap Group, 2001, p. 1047)

A disability is defined as: "A restriction or inability to perform an activity in the manner or within the range considered normal for a human being, mostly resulting from impairment" (Babotte, Grillemin, Nearkasen, & the Lorhandicap Group, 2001, p. 1047). Finally, WHO defines a handicap as: "This is the result of an impairment or disability that limits or prevents the fulfillment of one or several roles regarded as normal, depending on age, sex and social and cultural factors" (Babotte, Grillemin, Nearkasen, & the Lorhandicap Group, 2001, p. 1047).

Also there is the older definition of mental retardation by the German Council of Education, quoted by Beck and Konig (1994) as:

> A person is described as mentally retarded if, due to an organic-genetic or other impairment, his/her overall mental development and learning capacity is retarded to the extent that he/she likely will be in need of life-long social and educational support. The cognitive disability is often accompanied by those of the language, social, emotional, and motoric development. (p. 104)

Max would qualify under those two definitions as well. When it comes to developmental disabilities, there is a distinction of degree in Germany that roughly compares to the IQ limits of the AAMR definition. It includes persons with an IQ around 90 and some of the persons within the mild mental retardation group as learning disabled. The persons within the moderate and some of the persons from the severe mental retardation group in the U.S. would be classified as cognitive disabled in Germany, and some of the persons from the severe mental retardation group and the persons from the profound group would be identified as severely cognitive disabled. As it is not a general definition of degree, many professionals follow the American definition by AAMR and literally translate the categories. Learning disability is used as a milder form of cognitive disability that can be alleviated or corrected somewhat within the school system. Therefore the term "learning disability" is used in a different connotation in Germany than in the U.S.

Again, because there is not as much reliance on IQ tests in Germany, Max would be given a detailed diagnosis, and a disability profile (Behinderungsbild) would be established that includes the history of his disability as well as detailed information of the things he is or is not capable of. (For example, he can dress himself but needs help with shoelaces.) Such a disability profile would look similar to the description of

Max given in the introduction of the case example above. Max would most likely fall within the broader category of having a cognitive disability.

Early Detection

In Utero

Because Max's disability is not Down syndrome or a neural tube defect, it is unlikely that it would have been picked up by an Alpha Feto Protein (AFP) test. However, the heart defect and the slight spastic of his lower limbs could be picked up by ultrasound.

It is likely that his heart defect would be diagnosed earlier in Germany, because ultrasound examinations are part of every prenatal visit there. On the other hand, the disability might have been picked up by chorionic villius sampling (CVS) in the U.S. at a much earlier point, as tests like AFP and CVS are used much more extensively in the U.S. compared to Germany. However, it is not certain that either obstetrician/gynecologist would have noticed the disability in utero.

After the Birth of the Child

Both NRW and California have mandated newborn tests for disabilities. This makes it likely that the disability would have been picked up fairly soon after delivery. Because every person in Germany has mandatory health insurance, it is much more likely that Max would be evaluated on a continuous basis than it is in the U.S. However, Max's mother is a working mother with insurance that covers all the well-baby exams and inoculations. So Max's disability is first diagnosed on the 7th visit to the pediatrician in Germany and the U.S. (The initial diagnosis would be developmental delay because it is too early to specify all his difficulties.)

Orientation After Detection

After Max is diagnosed with a disability, his mother has to explore the different possibilities for his support and development. Assume she is very assertive and uses available services. When Max is 9 months of age, however, Max's mother in Germany has a valuable resource that his American mother does not have, and that is time.

Time and Money

The social safety net in Germany provides many preventive and safe-guard provisions for parents. For mothers who are employed, there are rules and regulations that have the safety and security of both the mother and child in mind. They are called Mutterschutz (mother safety). Among them are regulations on what kind of tasks she is allowed to do, at what times of the day and for how many hours she can work, and details regarding her paid leave from work (MuSCHG, §§ 1-24, 1997). Her paid leave starts 6 weeks before birth and ends 8 to 12 weeks after birth. After that time she can take something that is called Erzieungsurlaub (child-raising leave). This child-raising leave can last up to 36 months. During this entire time the employer cannot fire her and has to provide the same or an equal position, including equal pay, to her when she comes back to work. Also, her otherwise-accumulated vacation time from before her leave remains intact. The option of child-raising leave also exists for fathers. Parents can even take this leave together (BerzGG, §§ 1-24, 1985).

During the first 2 years of child-raising leave, the family receives Erzieungsgeld (child-raising money). At the time of this writing the amount is up to 300 Euro per child per month. In addition to this, every family receives Kindergeld (child money). It is paid for each child in the family and is usually provided until the child turns 18. If the child goes to college it can last until age 26. In case of a physical or intellectual disability that impedes the ability to earn a living wage, this money will be provided indefinitely. Currently the amount provided per child per month is 154 Euro. If there are more than three children, the amount for the additional children is a bit higher (EstG, §§ 62-78 aF. 2, 1997).

With these safeguards like job security, money, and child support from her husband in place, Max's mother in Germany decided early on that she would take two years off on child-raising leave. During this time she provides most of the care for her child. She also has her mother and her sister baby-sit him for sometimes, and she joins a toddler group when he is 6 months old.

Her American counterpart takes her two weeks of maternity leave before the birth of the child and her 6 weeks after. She receives child support from her ex-husband and relies heavily on her mother and sister for childcare in the first couple of months and day-care after the first 6 months. By the time Max is diagnosed, she has already been back to work full-time for quite some time.

Services

The first place for the California mom of Max to look for services is the Department of Developmental Services, and there she goes to one of the regional centers for local resources and services. In his case it would be the Frank D. Lanterman Regional Center. Max falls within the eligibility definition of section 95014 of the California Code as an infant and toddler, and later he qualifies under section 4512 of the California Welfare and Institutions code. This is the case because he has a significant developmental delay as an infant and toddler and is later diagnosed with mental retardation. Therefore the services provided by the regional center are free. There are several services offered at the center. Among them are information and referral, assessment and diagnosis, early intervention, and family support.

Assessment and Early Intervention

The procedure for Max and his mother to follow would be to bring him in for a thorough assessment first, at which time he would see as many specialists as necessary. For example, according to his needs he would see a neurologist, a cardiologist, and an orthopedic specialist. A case history would be established by a social worker, and the results of the individual examinations would be included to establish as complete a picture as possible.

On the basis of this assessment the social worker would then develop, together with Max's mother, an individualized family support plan (IFSP) and would do service coordination according to this plan. Once Max enters the school system the plan is called an individualized education plan (IEP). For now (at 9 months) it is not clear if the assessment can catch all the impairments that will eventually be discovered, as it is for some just too early to tell.

Early Intervention

The services that Max needs most at this point are the ones that are grouped under the term "early intervention." The early intervention program in California is called Early Start and is funded under part C of the Individuals with Disabilities Education Act Amendments of 1991 (IDEA; 1991). Information about all their services can be found on the Department of Disability Services website of the state of California (*http://www.dds.cahwnet.gov/*). Some of the services offered are assistive technology, counseling, occupational and physical therapy, social work services, and respite services. Parent-to-parent groups are also available.

The social worker and Max's mom will determine what services of those Max needs, if they are available in his area, and what services his mother can participate in on her tight schedule. Some of the services can also be provided with other relatives present, so that Max does not miss out on opportunities.

Medical Services

Services that do not fall under the regional centers' capabilities are ongoing medical services and supervision. For these Max has to see his pediatrician and the specialists that are needed for his care. Depending on the health insurance coverage of his mother, this will be a financially difficult task, and even under the best circumstances it will be a daunting task when it comes to scheduling those appointments. It will also be difficult for Max's mom to keep the specialists informed about what the other specialists are doing. Service coordination and case management services by the regional center can be somewhat helpful here. Last, Max has to change day-care settings because the day-care center he initially visits does not see itself equipped to respond to his disabilities.

In Germany Max also has access to early recognition and early intervention services. One of the places for his mother to go for information and referral services is the Deutsche Lebenshilfe ev. There she can find evaluation services and early intervention services that are similar to the ones offered in California at places called Fruehfoerderstellen (early support places). If she uses those, the several specialists will come to her home and provide services there (Antrettter, Koerner, & Mueller-Erichsen, 2002). If more concentrated efforts are required she can go to a Sozialpaedagogisches Zentrum (social-pedagogical center), where services are provided within the facility. Or she can use a combination of both. Disability-specific counseling and support groups are also available. She can go to the Sozialamt (social agency) and get counseling on all available services and eligibility requirements following the current laws. Almost all services and aids are covered by the social service system or health insurance.

As for day-care, there are several options, some segregated and some integrated. There are the possibilities to use day-mothers or -fathers (certified day-care providers who take one to three children into their homes during working hours), Kinderkrippen and Horte (places that specialize in the day-care of infant and toddlers), and toddler groups.

Max's mother decides on early intervention services within her home, and from the time she goes back to work until Max is 3 years old she arranges for a day-mother and has the early intervention team schedule visits at the day-mother's home as well as her own.

School Services

After Max turns 3 he can go to kindergarten (preschool). There are also segregated and integrated options there. He could be integrated as a child with a disability in a regular preschool, integrated with a group of other children with disabilities in a regular preschool, go to a special preschool where children without disabilities are integrated, go to a special preschool that shares facilities with a regular preschool, or go to a special preschool. However, not all options are available everywhere, and the idea of integration is not as established in Germany as it is in the U.S. Therefore he will go to a special preschool, as this is the most easily available option. Once he turns 6 years old Max transfers to a special school. This is currently the only option in NRW for school-aged children with developmental disabilities (Leske & Budrich, 2000).

There are a few model projects within the state, and a shift to more integrated offers are on the horizon. They have not become reality yet. Throughout the federation are also more integrated schooling options. Most of them are offered in the new states; those options include integration as the only child with a disability into a regular class or school (this option is mostly for children with physical disabilities only), being in a class with other students with disabilities in a regular school, cooperation among regular and special schools, and special boarding schools. All these options have in common that children with disabilities are still seen as more an exception in the regular school system than the rule. This view has been challenged in theory recently but has not changed much in practice settings. However, much care is taken to give students with disabilities the best education possible. This includes following individualized education plans and the integration of additional services like occupational therapy, physical therapy, and speech and language development within the curriculum. The newest teaching tools are used, and a teacher/student ratio of one-to-three or one-to-four exists.

Max's counterpart in the U.S. has much more integrated experiences in preschool and later in school. The IDEA act assures him an education in the least restrictive environment. In preschool he experiences integration with several other children with disabilities in a regular preschool. However, once he makes the transition to grade school, he is one of very few children with developmental disabilities in a regular school and the only one in his classroom. He participates with the help of a teacher's aide and gets pulled out for skills training some of the time. Also his mother learns that individual education plans are regarded differently by parents and schools and have to be ardently negotiated. The schools are faced with a tight budget, and some of Max's services have to be covered at home. Max's mother also has to arrange for alternative transportation to and from school, because Max gets lost easily when using regular school buses. By the time Max goes to grade school, his diagnosis is very much established and life has settled into a routine for him and his mother. The next big transition happens when Max finishes his schooling and decisions need to be made about where he will work and live in the future.

Transition Services and Options

In Germany Max goes to school as long as possible. He enjoys the company of his classmates, and his mother asks for extensions on his school stay to enhance his limited reading, writing, and counting abilities and to prepare him for his work in a supported employment facility. Two extensions are granted, and Max leaves school when he turns 18–the age of majority in Germany. At this point Max is regarded as an adult with all the rights and responsibilities of an adult without disabilities. However, he is not able to care for himself; therefore, social services together with his mother and him apply for a power of attorney (Betreung nach dem Betreuungsgesetz).

At this legal procedure it is determined what kind of support Max needs in his adult life when it comes to decision making and who should be the person who holds the power of attorney (BGB §§ 1896-1908 k, 2002). In Max's case the decision is easily made that he needs help in medical and economic decision making and that his mother will be his power of attorney. They get along well, and she is not restricting him in his decision-making processes but has always supported his independence. Sometimes these cases are not that simple, and a judge will appoint a guardian at litem during the determination procedure to keep the best interests of the person with the disability in mind. If it is determined that relatives do not qualify for the power of attorney position, one member from social services is appointed to take on the responsibility.

In any case, after a person turns 18, parents who have the power of attorney cannot assume that everything will go on as it has but must periodically check in with social services to assure that they handle their children's affairs in the best interest of their children. After a couple of years each case gets reevaluated to see if the supports provided are still needed by the person with the disability.

Max also decides that he will work in a supported employment facility, because most of his friends go there, and that he will move out from home into a small supported living facility. The decision about his work is one that also comes out of necessity, because Max is not able to partake in competitive employment and with a high unemployment rate in Germany, chances are slim for him to find any other job whatsoever. The decision to move away from home is supported by his mother and social services. Finding a space for him in a small supported living facility is a somewhat longer and harder process than he had expected.

About 60% of all adults with developmental disabilities live at home with their parents in Germany (Zirden, 2002). They receive Eingliederungshilfe, a disability-linked social service payment (BSHG, §§ 39-47, 1961). They also receive some money from their employment, although this is usually not enough to make a living. There are several other forms of living arrangements available; however, the more independent they are, the more rare they are to find.

For short periods of time (2 to 4 weeks a year) there is the possibility of Kurzzeitbetreuung (short-time supervision), where the adult is taken into an institution or nursing home and taken care of 24 hours a day. Eingliederungshilfe pays for this time in combination with health insurance and care insurance. This option is mostly seen as respite time for parents of persons with severe developmental disabilities.

Institutionalized living arrangements range in size and amount of supervision. There are group homes within institutions that have supervision all day. There are small groups available within apartments with full-time or part-time supervision. Also single apartments, couple apartments, and parent/children apartments with supervision are available. Eingliederungshilfe and social aid pay for all these living arrangements; the residents receive an allowance and do not manage monetary affairs like rent or board.

Independent living arrangements include living in apartments that are not connected to an institution. Those are available for single persons, couples, or groups of roommates. Some of these living arrangements include part-time supervision. Eingliederungshilfe and social aid also pay for them. However, independent living arrangements are much more flexible and have fairly new options to persons with disabilities.

After searching for a year, Max and his social worker find a space in an apartment with three roommates who have a caseworker come by twice a week for a couple of hours. Max likes to be around other people his age and considers himself lucky to have his new home and his job.

Max's counterpart in the U.S. graduates from high school at age 16 and tries to find a job in competitive employment. This is done together with his social worker and mother and some key persons in his life who form his support team, following the person-centered approach. He is a strong young man, good at sorting, and friendly to people. After a couple of setbacks he finds a job as a busboy at a restaurant. This work suits him because it is repetitive and he is among people. However, he does not want to do this for the rest of his life. The pay is not what he had expected, he gets easily overwhelmed at busy hours, and transportation to and from work is a problem. Also the employer hired him on a trial basis and cannot promise him any job security. He still lives at home, and neither he nor his mother are ready to change that yet. Max tries to confront work as a challenge he has to be familiar with before he wants to tackle the next step of living by himself. As for long-term plans, he is not sure what kind of a job and what kind of living arrangement he will have in the future.

CONCLUSION

This comparison highlights service options and living possibilities for persons with developmental disabilities in the U.S. and Germany. It seems to be the case that those options follow the theme of independence versus security. Services in the U.S. are not as easy to come by, and financial security is most of the time not given. The services that are available, however, usually have the most individualized and independent options available for the person with the disability. Supervision and guidance are not the most important issue; freedom of choice is. Even if the freedom of choice entails choosing not to be supported by anybody.

In Germany there are more services available, and it is important to not let anybody fall through the cracks. However, the range and scope of the service options are limited. In order to be able to provide services reliably to everybody, these services are more streamlined and less individualistic. Supervision and guidance are important. The word Betreuung includes both the meaning of supervision and guidance. It has a friendly connotation and comes close to the meaning of raising and caring for people. The aspect of helping and care-taking and close contact is something that is included in service provision. Nobody is left alone, as good or bad as that may be.

REFERENCES

Americans With Disabilities Act of 1990. (1990). Pub.L. No.101-336, 104 Stat. 327.

Antretter, R., Koerner, I., & Mueller-Erichsen, M. (2002). *Bundesvereinigung Lebenshilfe fuer Menschen mit geistiger Behinderung.* Retrieved September 7, 2002, from the World Wide Web: *http://www.lebenshilfe.de/.*

Babotte, E. Guillemin, F., Nearkasen, C., & Lorhandicap Group (2001). Prevalence of impairments, disabilities, handicaps, and quality of life in the general population: A review of recent literature. *Bulletin of the World Health Organization, 2001, 79,* (11).

Beck, I., & Konig, A. (1994). Quality of life for mentally retarded people in Germany: An overview of theory and practice. In D. Goode (Ed.), *Quality of life for persons with disabilities: International perspectives and issues* (pp. 103-125). Cambridge, MA: Brookline Books.

Berkowitz, E. (1987). *Disabled policy.* New York: Cambridge UP.

Betreunungsgesetz, Buergerliches Gesetzbuch 2002, §§ 1896-1908k. *BGBl. IS. 42 ber.S. 2909.*

Bundeserziehungsgeldgesetz, 1985, §§ 1-24. *BGBl I 1985, 2154.*

Bundessozialhilfegesetz, 1961, §§ 39-47. *BGBl I 1961, 815, 1875.*

California Department of Developmental Services Homepage. Retrieved September 9, 2002, from the World Wide Web: *http://www.dds.cahwnet.gov/.*

Developmental Disabilities Assistance and Bill of Rights Act of 1990. (1990). Pub.L. No. 101-496, 104 Stat. 1191.

Einkommenssteuergesetz, 1997, §§ 62-78 a.F.2. *BGBl. I 1997 S.2970.*

Individuals with Disabilities Education Act Amendments of 1991. (1991). Pub.L.No. 102-119, 105 Stat. 578.

Leske & Budrich's NRW-Lexikon.Politik.Gesellschaft.Wirtschaft.Recht.Kultur. (2nd ed.) (2000). Opladen, NRW: Verlag Leske & Budrich. Retrieved September 14, 2002 from the World Wide Web: *http://www.nrw.de/landnrw/nrwlex/lexschul.htm.*

Luckasson, R., Coulter, D. L., Polloway, E. A., Reiss, S., Schalock, R. L., Snell, M. E., Spitalnik, D. M., & Stark, J. A. (1992). *Mental retardation: Definition, classification, and systems of support* (9th ed.). Washington, DC: American Association on Mental Retardation.

Mutterschutzgesetz, 1997, §§ 1-24. *BGBl.I. S.22 ber. S.293.*

Zirden, H. (2002). *Wohnen fuer Behinderte.* Retrieved September 14, 2002 from the World Wide Web: *http://195.143.93.251/folgeseite_7020.html.*

Community Integration of Older People with Developmental Disabilities in Hong Kong

Raymond Man-hung Ngan
Mark Kin yin Li
Jacky Chau-kiu Cheung

Raymond Man-hung Ngan is Associate Head, Department of Applied Social Studies, City University of Hong Kong, Tat Chee Avenue, Kowloon Tong, Kowloon, Hong Kong.

Mark Kin-yin Li is Lecturer, Department of Social Work, Hong Kong Baptist University, University Road Campus, Kowloon Toong, Kowloon, Hong Kong.

Jacky Chau-kiu Cheung is Assistant Professor, Department of Applied Social Studies, City University of Hong Kong, Tat Chee Avenue, Kowloon Tong, Kowloon, Hong Kong.

The authors would like to thank Professors Carole and Alan Walker of the University of Sheffield (UK) for inspiring the Research Team to conduct a similar study in Hong Kong by their work in 1996, *Fair Shares for All? Disparities in Service Provision for Different Groups of People with Developmental Disabilities Living in the Community* (Brighton, UK: Pavilion). Moreover, the authors would like to express deepest gratitude to Professor Francis Yuen and the anonymous reviewer, who so kindly guided our revision of the manuscript.

Data from this study were obtained from a Strategic Research Grant funded by the City University of Hong Kong (CityU Project no: 7000819) and was published in a Research Report titled *Community Integration of Adults with Developmental Disabilities in Hong Kong* in July 2000 by the Department of Applied Social Studies, City University of Hong Kong. The Research Team was comprised of members Raymond Ngan, Mark Li, Jacky Cheung, Silva Yeung, and David Lok.

[Haworth co-indexing entry note]: "Community Integration of Older People with Developmental Disabilities in Hong Kong." Ngan, Raymond Man-hung, Mark Kin-yin Li, and Jacky Chau-kiu Cheung. Co-published simultaneously in *Journal of Social Work in Disability & Rehabilitation* (The Haworth Press, Inc.) Vol. 2, No. 2/3, 2003, pp. 101-119; and: *International Perspectives on Disability Services: The Same But Different* (ed: Francis K. O. Yuen) The Haworth Press, Inc., 2003, pp. 101-119. Single or multiple copies of this article are available for a fee from The Haworth Document Delivery Service [1-800-HAWORTH, 9:00 a.m. - 5:00 p.m. (EST). E-mail address: docdelivery@haworthpress.com].

http://www.haworthpress.com/store/product.asp?sku=J198
10.1300/J198v02n02_07

SUMMARY. To understand the community integration of adults with developmental disabilities in Hong Kong, a comprehensive measure includes four dimensions, pertaining to social activity, social services, interpersonal behavior, and people involved in social interaction. Applying this measure to 692 adults (aged 15-62), the territory-wide study finds that these adults lack company for out-of-home activities and community activities despite their higher knowledge, assertiveness, social interaction, and feeling accepted in the community. With the strengthening of many conditions (including knowledge and community support) for community integration, the adults tend to have greater need for empowerment to enhance their active participation in community activities. *[Article copies available for a fee from The Haworth Document Delivery Service: 1-800-HAWORTH. E-mail address: <docdelivery@haworthpress.com> Website: <http://www.HaworthPress.com> © 2003 by The Haworth Press, Inc. All rights reserved.]*

KEYWORDS. Community integration, developmental disability, assertiveness, feeling accepted, family protection, cooperation

Nowadays more people with mental disabilities are surviving into their old age due to improvements in medical science and living standards. Probably, these older people may be in double jeopardy, which implies increased community resistance, due to the developmental disability and old age (Walker, Walker, & Ryan, 1996). As such, they may not receive appropriate assistance because of the prominence of negative stereotypes about intellectual decline and physical disability associated with old age. Nevertheless, it is important to tap these people's experience of double jeopardy to clarify how various social institutions, service providers, and communities understand and treat these older people.

In Hong Kong (now a Special Administrative Region of China), encouraging people with disabilities to live in the community has been the fundamental objective in developing services for people with developmental disabilities since 1977 (Hong Kong Government, 1977). Policymakers acknowledge these people's rights to community integration, normalization, social-life valorization in developing Program Plans and Service White Papers for them (Hong Kong Government, 1992, 1995, 1997). However, obstacles–notably resistance and discrimination that these people encounter in the community–still exist and affect their levels of community integration (Lau & Cheung, 1999; Tse, 1994a, 1994b). Other conditions compromising their successful integration in the community may include aging, lack of knowledge, and social skills in the part of adults with developmental disabilities (Walker, Ryan, & Walker, 1996). The impact of age on the community integration of these adults has been a neglected area in research and policy (Walker, Ryan, & Walker, 1996).

Despite the emphasis on community integration since 1977, there has not been a comprehensive, territory-wide, systematic, and coherent evaluative study on the patterns, problems, and actual experiences of adults with developmental disabilities in Hong Kong. It is in light of this background and prior research in the United Kingdom (Walker et al., 1996) that the present study emerges to ascertain these people's experiences of community integration in Hong Kong (Ngan, Cheung, Yeung, Li, & Lok, 2000).

DEFINITION OF COMMUNITY INTEGRATION AND THE CONCEPTUAL FRAMEWORK

The present study goes beyond a typical conceptualization of community integration of adults with developmental disabilities as participation in community activities (Walker, Ryan, & Walker, 1996). Specifically, earlier research regarded the adults' use of services of hairdressing, banking, cinemas, theaters, restaurants, pubs, places of worship, sport, social clubs, and libraries as instances of community integration (Walker, Ryan, & Walker, 1996). With closer examination, these instances reveal that community integration broadly encompasses such dimensions as social interaction, relationship with family and friends, awareness of and participation in community activities, work, leisure activities, motivation toward living in a community, socialization, and communication (Schalock & Kiernan, 1990). Accurate portrayals of these various forms of community integration can offer an adequate understanding of the actual patterns and problems experienced by adults with developmental disabilities.

Community integration thus conceptually includes the following dimensions: (a) social activity, (b) social services, (c) interpersonal behavior, and (d) people involved in social interaction (see Figure 1). Each dimension in turn comprises a number of indicators (Ngan et al., 2000). The dimension of social activity, for instance, has the following indicators for measurement: social interaction, the availability of company, knowledge of the community, assertiveness, being accepted, desire for activity, and a low amount of family protection. Indicators related to social services are knowledge, use of, and the need for social services. The dimension of interpersonal behavior comprises the following indicators: cooperation and trouble making. Four types of people–children, youth, middle-aged adults, and older adults (defined by respondents)–represent different partners for social interaction and conversation as experienced by adults with developmental disabilities. In all, questions concerning the indicators employed wording shown in Tables 2, 3, 4,

FIGURE 1. Conceptual Framework of Community Integration

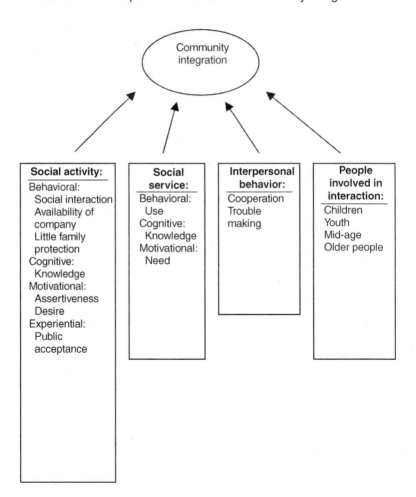

and 5. Respondents provide answers to the dimensions of social activity, social service, and partnership, whereas interviewers give ratings on the interpersonal behavior of adults with developmental disabilities.

METHODS

The study employed a three-stage approach composed of focus group discussion before and after a territory-wide survey of adults (aged 15 and above) with developmental disabilities. The focus groups served two major functions. Before the large-scale survey, initial focus groups respectively consisting of parents of adult children with developmental disabilities and social workers in both residential and community-based services helped gather relevant dimensions and indicators to prepare for appropriate measuring instruments for the survey. Consequently, the focus groups after the community-wide survey served to elaborate, corroborate, and explain results obtained from the survey (Morgan, 1996).

In all, the study covered a span of 1.5 years in 1998-99 to collect data successively from two focus groups of parents and professional social workers, followed by a survey of 692 adults with developmental disabilities, and last with another two focus groups composed of parents and professional social workers again. The quantitative and qualitative data collected contributed to the thorough investigation of the subject matter.

The community-wide survey collected data from a representative sample of 692 adults with developmental disabilities through the assistance of 55 service units in Hong Kong from 1998 to June 1999. The service units, affiliated with 13 agencies, provided various services, including residential, day care, work, training, and recreational services to people with intellectual disabilities.

The design purposively sampled proportionately more people with a severe grade of developmental disabilities to capture enough variance for the small group. As a result, 17.2% of the sample were adults with a severe grade of developmental disabilities, 49.4% being those with a moderate grade, and 33.4% with a mild grade (see Table 1). However, data from the census in 1999 showed that there were about 135,378 people with developmental disabilities, among them 116,620 being in the mild grade, 13,720 in the moderate grade, 4,802 in the severe grade, and 2,058 in the profound grade, based on the DSM-III classification (Hong Kong Government, 1999). In order to make the present study best represent the distribution of the three grades (from mild to severe) in the total

TABLE 1. Percentage of Sample Characteristics (*N* = 692)

		Unweighted %	Weighted %
Mental handicap	Mild	33.4	86.3
	Moderate	49.4	10.2
	Severe	17.2	3.6
Age	15-19	8.5	10.7
	20-29	33.1	33.4
	30-39	35.1	35.5
	40-49	18.8	17.0
	50-59	3.8	2.8
	60+	0.8	0.5
Sex	Male	49.7	51.2
	Female	50.3	48.8
Having a spouse	No	92.0	93.6
	Yes	8.0	6.4
Hostel residence	No	42.4	58.4
	Yes	57.6	41.6

population of people with developmental disabilities in Hong Kong, a weighting procedure served to weigh cases of the three grades to reflect the distribution in the population. After the weighting, the percentage of adults with the severe grade was 3.6%, that of adults with the moderate grade, 10.2%, and last, 86.3% for adults with the mild grade of developmental disabilities (see Table 1).

The study gathered data primarily from adults with developmental disabilities. In case it was not feasible to obtain information from them for every question item, the study relied on proxy responses from the family members or service providers of adults participating in the study. Among responses to items concerning community integration, on average 6.10% came from family members and 3.28% came from social workers. To avoid overestimating or underestimating from proxy responses, the study identified by regression analysis the difference between proxy responses and self-reports and used this to adjust for the scores of proxy responses. Practically, regression coefficients estimated from indicators for proxy responses identified the adjustment factor. Hence, if the proxy respondent reported a consistently higher score than that reported by the target respondent, the score should become lower. These adjusted scores were the basis for subsequent analysis.

Among the 692 sampled adults with developmental disabilities, about half (50.3%) consisted of female people. The respondents were primarily in the age group between 20 and 39 years. The average person was 32.1 years, but about one quarter (23.4%) of the sample was aged 40 and above. Slightly over half (57.6%) of the respondents lived in residential homes. Only 8.0% of all respondents had spouses.

RESULTS

Levels of Community Integration

Modest Level of Social Interaction. Despite the emphasis on full participation and equal opportunities (Hong Kong Government, 1992), social interaction among adults with developmental disabilities was only at a moderate level, with a mean of 58.8 on a 0-100 scale (see Table 2), weighted for the population of adults with developmental disabilities in Hong Kong. Adjusted for proxy responses, the mean was 59.6, which was at a similar moderate level. This figure would indicate the average level of social interaction if all data came directly from adults with developmental disabilities in Hong Kong.

Social interaction was least likely in terms of going to a new place. Only 27.1% of adults with developmental disabilities went to a new place in the month before the survey. Going to a recreation club (adjusted mean = 35.8), going outside with others to play (adjusted mean = 44.7), and going to a bank (adjusted mean = 45.6) were other less common forms of social interaction. Social interaction in terms of working with others to accomplish something and talking with neighbors was also at a moderate level, with adjusted means of 58.4 and 54.2 respectively.

Nevertheless, social interaction scores appeared higher in terms of use of public transportation. The adjusted mean for the adults was an 89.1 score, which stood out at a high level on a 0-100 scale. Second, dining with colleagues was the next most common form of social interaction, with an adjusted mean of 78.6.

Lack of Company in Going Out. The adults' desire for community integration was on average high, with an adjusted mean of 76.5, notably with the desire for going to a park and going to a playground to do exercise, with adjusted means of 74.7 and 73.9 respectively (Ngan et al., 2000). However, this strong desire of going out for activities did not correspond with the availability of company in going out. The availabil-

TABLE 2. Percent and Means Regarding Social Interaction

	% No	% Not sure	% Yes	Mean	Mean adjusted[a] for no proxy response
1. Taking public transportation vehicles	11.7	0.5	87.9	88.1	89.1
2. Dining with colleagues	21.7	1.4	76.9	77.6	78.6
3. Going to eat or buy at a fast food restaurant	23.2	1.4	75.4	76.1	75.7
4. Participating in activities of the center, hostel, or workshop	26.3	2.2	71.5	72.6	73.6
5. Talking with friends	28.2	1.4	70.4	71.1	72.3
6. Working with others to accomplish a thing	42.7	2.6	54.8	56.1	58.4
7. Talking with neighbors	46.3	2.6	51.0	52.3	54.2
8. Going to a bank	56.2	1.4	42.4	43.1	**45.6**
9. Going outside with others to play	52.2	0.9	46.9	47.3	**44.7**
10. Going to a recreational club	65.3	1.3	33.4	34.1	**35.8**
11. Going to a new place	69.4	3.5	27.1	28.9	**27.7**
Average social interaction score				58.8	59.6

[a]*Note.* The adjusted mean was the mean under the condition that all responses would come from the adults with mental handicaps themselves. It was adjusted for the amount of overreport or underreport due to proxy response.

ity of a partner in going to a playground or a community center was at a low level, with adjusted means of 40.7 and 36.9 respectively (see Table 3).

Fair Knowledge of the Community. The level of knowledge about the community among the adults was at a moderate to fair level, with an unadjusted mean of 59.7 and an adjusted mean of 62.3 for no proxy response (see Table 4). Findings of particular concern to policymakers and service administrators are as follows:

1. Less than one third (29.2%) of the adults knew how to go to a recreational club.
2. Less than half of the adults possessed knowledge to go to the following places: (a) knowing how to participate in activities of community centers (42.6%), (b) knowing how to see a doctor (46.4%), and (c) knowing how to go to a playground to do exercise (47.4%).

TABLE 3. Percent and Means Regarding the Availability of Company

	% No	% Not sure	% Yes	Mean	Mean adjusted for no proxy response
1. Having a good friend	20.9	1.7	77.4	78.3	81.6
2. Having someone going with you to play outside	44.7	0.4	54.9	55.1	53.5
3. Having someone going with you going to a playground to do exercise	57.3	1.3	11.4	42.1	40.7
4. Having someone going with you to a community center	61.0	1.5	37.4	38.2	36.9
Average				53.4	53.2

TABLE 4. Percent and Means Regarding Knowledge About the Community

	% No	% Not sure	% Yes	Mean	Mean adjusted for no proxy response
1. Knowing how to make a better outlook	20.3	3.0	76.7	78.2	80.2
2. Knowing how to buy at a supermarket	24.3	1.0	74.7	75.2	77.8
3. Knowing how to participate in activities of the center, hostel, or workshop	27.0	2.8	70.2	71.6	75.2
4. Knowing how to go to a park	31.7	1.0	67.3	67.8	69.5
5. Knowing how to make friends	33.8	3.2	63.1	64.6	68.6
6. Knowing how to go to an emporium	35.1	1.1	63.8	64.3	66.5
7. Knowing how to go for tea	36.4	1.5	62.1	62.9	66.0
8. Familiarity with neighbors	31.5	5.1	63.4	65.9	66.0
9. Knowing how to go outside	38.0	0.3	61.7	61.8	64.1
10. Knowing how to go to a bank	45.5	1.7	52.8	53.7	57.6
11. Knowing how to go to a playground to do exercise	50.3	2.3	47.4	48.5	51.8
12. Knowing how to see a doctor	52.5	1.1	46.4	46.9	49.5
13. Knowing how to participate in activities of community centers	55.4	2.0	42.6	43.6	46.4
14. Knowing how to go to a recreational club	68.4	2.4	29.2	30.4	32.5
Average mean				59.7	62.3

A Moderate Level of Assertiveness. Assertiveness hereby referred to the case that the adult dared to try out something on his or her own effort. Overall speaking, their assertiveness was at a moderate level, with a mean of 53.0 (see Table 5). The highest level of assertiveness manifested in terms of their own daring to make friends with others, with an adjusted mean of 63.7. The next highest assertiveness was in their daring to go outside alone, with an adjusted mean of 56.3. On the other hand, their daring to go to see a doctor alone was the lowest (mean = 44.5 among items indicative of assertiveness). These findings show that the adults might have the least difficulty in making friends. However, they dared not to see doctors, probably because they were afraid to receive medical treatment.

A High Level of Perception of Being Accepted in the Community. It was found that the adults expressed a high level of being accepted in the community, with an adjusted mean of 80.6 (see Table 6). There was no significant difference in the overall feeling of being accepted among adults of different grades of mental retardation. Only in the item concerning feeling of being well served in taking public transportation was there a significant difference. In this regard, adults of the severe grade felt the least acceptance from public transportation service (59.5 versus 87.5 scores for the mild grade). Another item (being well served in retail shops) also manifested a statistically significant difference. Adults of the severe grade showed the lowest adjusted mean (66.3), as opposed to the adjusted mean (80.9) for their mild grade counterparts.

Community Integration Being Inadequate and Adequate in Different Areas. Adults with developmental disabilities showed both adequate

TABLE 5. Percent and Means Regarding Assertiveness

	% No	% Not sure	% Yes	Mean	Mean adjusted for no proxy response
1. Daring to make friends with others alone	37.3	3.7	39.0	60.9	63.7
2. Daring to go outside alone	43.9	1.9	54.2	55.1	56.3
3. Daring to participate in activities in community centers alone	53.2	2.5	44.3	45.5	47.3
4. Daring to go to see a doctor alone	56.3	2.9	40.6	42.1	44.5
Average				51.0	53.0

TABLE 6. Weighted and Adjusted Means of Summary Scores of Community Integration and Empowerment

	Mild	Moderate	Severe	Overall
Social activity				
Social interaction	59.5	61.4	10.2	59.6
Availability of company	52.6	58.6	51.4	53.2
Knowledge of the community	64.3	52.7	40.8	62.3
Assertiveness	55.4	40.1	32.6	53.0
Feeling of being accepted	80.7	80.6	78.6	80.6
Desire for community integration	76.6	76.7	75.7	76.5
Family protection	45.7	49.6	35.5	45.8
Social services				
Knowledge of social services	42.9	31.2	31.8	41.5
Use of social services	23.3	23.6	27.1	23.5
Need for social services	51.9	51.4	48.9	51.7
Inadequate use relative to need	8.7	5.9	12.0	8.6
Interpersonal behavior				
Cooperation	66.7	67.0	64.4	66.7
Trouble making	6.1	9.7	14.0	6.5
Partnership				
Talking most with children	7.7	5.4	5.1	6.2
Talking most with youth	25.8	13.1	7.6	17.2
Talking most with middle age adults	51.7	56.9	67.1	56.4
Talking most with older adults	14.9	24.6	20.3	20.3

and inadequate community integration, but in different areas. Their experience of being accepted by people in the community was high, but their use of social services was mostly inadequate (23.5 on a 0-100 scale in the use of rehabilitation bus service in the recent month versus 51.7 on such needs). A mean deficit score of 19.1 registered the need for adult education service.

While the great majority of the adults had the experience of taking public transportation, dining with colleagues, and going to eat at a fast food restaurant, few had gone to a new place or a recreational club. Participation was not adequate in going outside with reliable company to play and going to a bank. Because recreation and play tend to be essential activities to them (Putnam, Werder, & Schleien, 1985), deficiency in these items would be particularly undesirable for their community integration. Besides, the availability of company (mean = 53.2), assertiveness (mean = 53.0), and knowledge about the community (mean = 62.3) showed a similar modest level of community integration that would not appear to be very satisfactory to their parents. Although their adult children expressed a very strong desire of going out (mean = 76.5) and visits by volunteers (mean score = 85.6), they suffered from a lack of company to do so.

EMPOWERING OLDER PEOPLE WITH DEVELOPMENTAL DISABILITIES FOR COMMUNITY INTEGRATION

To address the question about differences in the level of community integration between the older adults (aged 45 or above) and those younger adults aged between 15 and 44, multivariate statistical analysis controlled for a number of background characteristics to provide proper tests and estimates. Results show that older adults tended to have (a) relatively less chance to have company for community activities; (b) poor knowledge and lesser use of social services regardless of a larger need; (c) lower assertiveness, especially for those living in institutions, and (d) deficient social interaction.

Relatively Less Chance to Have Company for Community Activities

Older people (aged 45+) were relatively less likely than their younger counterparts (aged between 15 and 29) to have company in going out (mean = 55.7 vs. 58.8). A general pattern emerged: the older the age of the respondents, the lesser the likelihood to have company (see Table 7). This pattern is undesirable to older adults with developmental disabilities, as explained by parents participating in the focus group: "People with developmental disabilities are poor in social skills. As a result, it is difficult for them to make friends and find companions and to stand on their own feet when they grow up. They are unable to participate in most social circles, except those organized in a community center."

In contrast, focus group interviews indicated that whereas the professionals (social workers) were optimistic about the community integration of adults with developmental disabilities, their parents had a reservation about it. In support of their views, professionals were able to mention a number of incidents indicative of the community integration,

TABLE 7. Adjusted Means by Age Group

	15-29	30-44	45+
Cooperation	65.6	66.3	64.2
Trouble making	**7.8**	**11.0**	**12.9**
Assertiveness	41.6	43.3	41.3
Availability of company	**58.8**	**48.9**	**55.7**
Feeling accepted	79.8	80.2	79.1
Desire for activity	77.5	75.6	71.3
Social interaction	**62.4**	**55.0**	**58.6**
Community knowledge	54.8	50.7	50.9
Family protection	**46.7**	**42.8**	**37.6**
Being brought outside by the family	**62.2**	**58.0**	**44.5**
Knowledge of social services	38.6	33.8	27.0
Use of social services	27.1	22.2	24.8
Need for social services	50.7	48.0	57.6

Note. Boldface figures indicated significant difference at .05 level.

such as "they often visit elderly homes and hospitals" and "they have high desire to go to youth centers and participate in activities there. As a result of going there, they would experience a lot of new stimuli." Parents tended to have great reservations regarding their children's abilities. They were afraid their children might hurt others as well as being hurt. They chose to protect their grown-up children and keep a close eye on them. Thus, the older adults with developmental disabilities were having relatively less chance to have their families bring them (means of 44.5 for aged 45+, 58.0 for the age group of 30-44, and 62.2 for those aged 15-29; see Table 7). Hence, it is desirable to nourish the parents' faith in their adult children's abilities for community education.

Poor Knowledge and Lesser Use of Social Services, Regardless of a Larger Need

Table 7 shows that older people with developmental disabilities tended to have relatively poor knowledge of social services than did their younger counterparts (means = 27.0 vs. 38.6). Despite older people's stronger need for social services (mean = 57.6 on a scale from 0 to 100), their use of such services was at a low level (mean = 24.8). Focus group interviews found that whereas the professionals affirmed the effectiveness and helpfulness of most social services, the parents had a reservation about this. A crucial reason was that the parents had only sporadic and limited experience with social services. Views expressed by parents were as follows:

1. "People working with the hostel seldom bring the residents outside."
2. "The sheltered workshop does not provide much assistance to people there. People just fight among each other in the workshop with no one's care."
3. "It is difficult for people with developmental disabilities to go outside without rehabilitation bus service."

It is therefore necessary to pinpoint where the gaps between perceptions of the professionals and parents were. Apparently, much of the parents' reservation tended to stem from rumors about the services. As such, the parents would require proper knowledge about the services, which in turn hinges on their direct experience with the use of the services.

Lower Assertiveness, Especially for Those Living in Institutions

Compared with the younger adults, older adults with developmental disabilities appeared to have relatively lower assertiveness, which referred to daring to try out something on their own effort (see Table 7). For the age group of 45 or above, the adjusted mean of assertiveness was 55.7, which was relatively lower than the mean (58.8) for the younger group (aged between 15 and 29). In particular, those older adults aged 45 or above living in institutions reported a much lower assertiveness score (mean = 35.0) when compared with their counterparts living in community (mean = 63.9) (see Table 8). This is a matter of concern to professionals working with them in institutions because they should be aware of the need to improve the community living and socialization skills of their clients. Moreover, the older adults also suffered from a relatively deficient and lower score on knowledge about the community and social services (mean = 47.8 from the hostel sample versus 62.5 for the same age group living in community). When confronted with these findings, professional social workers in focus group interviews explained that there was a lack of staffing in social services and that they had to work in shifts in institutions. Fundamentally, there seems to be a lack of sufficient trained social work personnel in homes for the mentally disabled.

TABLE 8. Adjusted Means by Age Group by Dwelling Type

	Family dwelling			Hostel dwelling		
	15-29	30-44	45+	15-29	30-44	45+
Assertiveness	**37.9**	**40.0**	**63.9**	**48.3**	**45.8**	**35.0**
Social interaction	**61.2**	**53.4**	51.8	59.2	59.8	59.1
Community knowledge	52.2	48.6	**62.5**	55.1	54.7	47.8
Family protection	41.9	**54.4**	36.2	44.1	39.8	35.3
Use of social services	27.3	21.5	26.0	21.2	25.0	25.7
Need for social services	**52.4**	39.0	**67.6**	47.1	**57.6**	46.6

Note. Boldface figures indicated significant difference at .05 level.

Deficient Social Interaction

Table 7 shows that the older adults (aged 45+) tended to have relatively lower scores on social interaction in the community (mean = 58.6 versus 62.4 for the youngest age group). Besides, interviewers of the older adults tended to report significantly higher scores on trouble-making behavior (adjusted mean = 12.9 versus 7.8 for the youngest age group). It seems that their skills to improve social interaction and effective socialization skills need further empowerment by professionals working with them, in community-based services, domiciliary training services, and residential homes.

DISCUSSION

Community Integration: From Normalization to Empowerment

In Hong Kong, community integration has been the fundamental objective in developing services for people with disabilities, including developmental disabilities, since 1977. After almost 24 years of implementation, it is timely to move the hitherto policy emphasis from normalization, social rights, and community acceptance to empowering effective skills for older people with developmental disabilities toward their active participation in the community. There is a strong demand for more inclusive models of care for people with developmental disabilities, especially to fulfill the strong desire of older adults for community participation as shown by data in the present study. These people's voices should deserve public attention, as it has been increasing so in the British context (Walker, Ryan, & Walker, 1996).

Walker and Walker (1998) pointed out that the adoption of normalization as a model of support for people with developmental disabilities indicates that, in principle, the "heart is in the right place." However, they commented that it is problematic in its operationalization, and this is so, largely, because service providers and others are falling into the trap of equating the needs of the older adults to those of the younger. Besides, there is another misconception that older people with developmental disabilities should gradually withdraw from everyday community life and confine themselves in institutions. Findings from the present study show the need for dispelling the discriminatory stereotype. It is necessary to attend to the strong desire of older adults with developmental disabilities for community activities and companions. Service provision should cater to these people's needs rather than to the original structure of services (Walker, Ryan, & Walker, 1996).

Older people with developmental disabilities, however, do not have sufficient skills for community inclusion. Data from the present study show that their assertiveness and social interaction were particular areas in need of improvement because of their low levels (means = 53.0 and 53.2). In particular, promotion of assertiveness skills for adults with severe developmental disabilities and those older adults residing in institutions is especially necessary (means = 32.6 and 35.0). To start with, it is necessary to promote their participation in a recreational club (mean = 35.8). It is also necessary to facilitate their participation by providing them with company in going out. This is crucial because their social interaction and the availability of company are inadequate, which is a problem in the United Kingdom as well (Walker, Ryan, & Walker, 1996).

Walker and Walker (1998) asserted that the creation of a supportive environment would provide the framework for addressing the social integration of older people with developmental disabilities. Our findings reveal that at times parents were overprotective and prohibited their adult children from going out and talking with strangers out of a fear that they would probably be hurt or looked down upon. However, the older adults reported that they were seldom brought outside by their families (mean = 44.5). It is therefore necessary to mitigate the overprotective atmosphere inside the family. Parents should realize the actual assertive abilities of their adult children.

Professionals in focus group interviews emphasized the usefulness of empowerment training for their adult clients with developmental disabilities. However, they admitted that they at present suffer from a lack of sufficient trained personnel to develop active empowerment training courses and group activities for community living skills to promote the assertiveness and social interaction skills of their clients. Domiciliary training services would now appear essential empowering tools to strengthen the level of community integration for older people with developmental disabilities. Fundamentally, development of empowering skills for community integration would allow effective community integration of older people with developmental disabilities in recognition of their strong desire for inclusion in the community. It is essential that service providers do not create additional barriers by inappropriate age stereotyping.

Limitations

Admittedly, measurement of the community integration of people with developmental disabilities may contain biases. Although the biases may clearly stem from such sources as the respondents' understanding of questions, desire to present socially desirable answers, and to perpetuate support from social services (Edgerton, 1993; Wilhite & Sheldon, 1997), the effects of these biases are not transparent. The difficulty rests in the case that these biases may not affect all responses and all respondents consistently and systematically in an expected manner. There does not seem to be a way to eliminate this trouble by relying exclusively on the self- or proxy report. The only way toward valid measurement is to employ multiple measures, incorporating self-report, proxy report, observation, and other tracking mechanisms together. Nevertheless, the integration of multiple measures is vulnerable to additional biases and confounding factors such as the availability of service and opportunity of participation, and the influence of service providers. The integrated measure may no longer reflect the genuine free will of the individual. Thus, the integrated measures need not supplant the self-report, which is a valuable measure of the individual's voice.

CONCLUSION

With the caveat that there may be biases in self- and proxy report and minor variation due to proxy report, data show that adults with developmental disabilities in Hong Kong tend to enjoy adequate community integration in terms of feeling accepted, social interaction in public facilities, having friends, and knowledge about daily living. Their community integration, nonetheless, is lower in terms of the availability of company and social interaction and knowledge regarding specific activities and services. Such inadequacy within a rather supportive community calls for more empowerment for the adults' better use of facilities and social services in the community.

REFERENCES

Edgerton, R. B. (1993). *The cloak of competence.* Berkeley: University of California Press.

Hong Kong Government. (1977). *Integrating the disabled into the community: A united effort* (white paper). Hong Kong: Author.

Hong Kong Government. (1992). *Green paper by the Working Party on Rehabilitation Policies and Services on Equal Opportunities and Full Participation.* Hong Kong: Author.

Hong Kong Government. (1995). *White paper on rehabilitation policies for the disabled.* Hong Kong: Author.

Hong Kong Government. (1997). *Programme plan review on services for the disabled in Hong Kong.* Hong Kong: Health and Welfare Branch, Government Secretariat.

Hong Kong Government. (1999). *Programme plan review on services for the disabled in Hong Kong.* Hong Kong: Health and Welfare Branch, Government Secretariat.

Lau, J., & Cheung, J. (1999). Factors associated with discriminatory attitudes towards mentally retarded persons and psychiatric patients. *International Social Work, 42,* 431-444.

Morgan, D. L. (1996). Focus groups. *Annual Review of Sociology, 22,* 129-152.

Ngan, R., Cheung, J., Yeung, S., Li, M., & Lok, D. (2000). *Community integration of adults with mental handicaps in Hong Kong: Research report.* Hong Kong: Department of Applied Social Studies, City University of Hong Kong.

Putnam, J.W., Werder, J.K., & Schleien, S.J. (1985). Leisure and Recreation Services for Handicapped Persons. In K.C. Lakin & R.H. Bruininks (Eds.), Strategies for achieving community integration of developmentally disabled citizens (pp. 253-276). Baltimore, MD: Brookes.

Schalock, R. L., & Kiernan, W. E. (1990). *Habilitation planning for adults with disabilities.* New York: Springer-Verlag.

Tse, J. (1994a). Community resistance to mental handicap facilities in Hong Kong. *British Journal of Developmental Disabilities, 22,* 100-103.

Tse, J. (1994b). Discriminating against people with mental retardation in Hong Kong. *International Social Work, 37,* 357-368.

Walker, A., & Walker, C. (1998). Normalisation and normal ageing: The social construction of dependency among older people with learning disabilities. *Disability & Society, 13,* 125-142.

Walker, A., Walker, C., & Ryan, T. (1996). Older people with developmental disabilities leaving institutional care: A case of double jeopardy. *Ageing & Society, 16,* 1-26.

Walker, C., Ryan, T., & Walker, A. (1996). *Fair shares for all? Disparities in service provision for different groups of people with developmental disabilities living in the community.* Brighton, UK: Pavilion.

Wilhite, B., & Sheldon, K. (1997). Consumer satisfaction for individuals with developmental disabilities. *Activities, Adaptation & Aging, 21,* 71-77.

Hmong Americans' Changing Views and Approaches Towards Disability: Shaman and Other Helpers

Serge C. Lee

Francis K. O. Yuen

SUMMARY. This article discusses how the concept of disability has evolved among Hmong Americans. The term disability has its unique cultural roots in Hmong traditions. Findings from a study of a sample of Hmong Americans in Northern California confirm the changing Hmong Americans' views on the issue of disability and their use of shaman. Families, community leaders, and shaman continue to be the primary support network and sources of consultation for many Hmong Americans. *[Article copies available for a fee from The Haworth Document Delivery Service. 1-800-HAWORTH. E-mail address: <docdelivery@haworthpress.com> Website: <http://www.HaworthPress.com> © 2003 by The Haworth Press, Inc. All rights reserved.]*

KEYWORDS. Hmong Americans, shaman, disability, cultural beliefs

Serge C. Lee is Associate Professor, Division of Social Work, California State University-Sacramento, Sacramento, CA 95819-6090.

Francis K. O. Yuen is Professor, Division of Social Work, California State University-Sacramento, Sacramento, CA 95819-6090.

[Haworth co-indexing entry note]: "Hmong Americans' Changing Views and Approaches Towards Disability: Shaman and Other Helpers." Lee, Serge C., and Francis K. O. Yuen. Co-published simultaneously in *Journal of Social Work in Disability & Rehabilitation* (The Haworth Press, Inc.) Vol. 2, No. 2/3, 2003, pp. 121-132; and: *International Perspectives on Disability Services: The Same But Different* (ed: Francis K. O. Yuen) The Haworth Press, Inc., 2003, pp. 121-132. Single or multiple copies of this article are available for a fee from The Haworth Document Delivery Service [1-800-HAWORTH, 9:00 a.m. - 5:00 p.m. (EST). E-mail address: docdelivery@haworthpress.com].

10.1300/J198v02n02_08

Beyond the official and legal definitions, disability is a relative concept and condition that is subject to different interpretations within the given sociocultural contexts. Indigenous people from homogeneous societies may have rather unique and different perspectives toward disability in comparison to those in a heterogeneous and jurisprudent society such as the United States.

Hmong American is an ethnic group of people who were primarily farmers living in the mountainous areas of northern Laos, a small Southeast Asian country. Indigenous people from the southwestern region of China migrated into the mountain of Laos in the early 19th century. They lived a relatively simple, tranquil, and hardworking agricultural life style (Hamilton-Merritt, 1993; Mottin, 1980; Quincy, 1988). Formal education was not common among these uncomplicated native people. Except for the French and American involvement in Southeast Asia, the Hmong were relatively unknown to the outside world. It was only after the Vietnam War that the word "Hmong" began to appear more in Western literature and in some of the major Western dictionaries or thesauruses.

Hmong Americans arrived in the United States in large numbers after the Vietnam War in the late 1970s and early 1980s. It was estimated that 150,000 Hmong arrived as refugees to the United States during those years (Vang, 2001). In 2000, the U.S Census Bureau put the Hmong population at 169,428 (http://www.hmongstudies.org/50statbyrani.html). However, most Hmong disagreed with the census figure. Some believed that since most of them came from Laos and originally they were known as Laotian Hmong, some might continue to call themselves Laotian. With the Hmong people continuing the tradition of a moderate family size, it is estimated that the Hmong American population has doubled in the last 2.5 decades. The best estimate put the total Hmong American population at 300,000 (Vang, 2001).

Acculturating into the U.S. society while preserving their traditional culture and virtue are the day-to-day challenges for many Hmong families. On a similar note, developing culturally competent practice has been the main thrust for the social work profession in the past two decades. Many have written about the different aspects of culturally specific practice with Asian Americans. For many practical and historical reasons, most of these writings have been on Chinese, Japanese, or Korean Americans–the largest Asian groups that have a longer history in the United States.

Recent papers on practice with Southeast Asian refugee populations also fall into the same population-size limitation and have focused

mostly on larger groups such as Vietnamese and Cambodians. Literature searches using reputable academic on-line databases revealed that
Hmong Americans have not been the focus of academic papers, particularly in social work. LexisNexis identified 286 news articles on Hmong
Americans between August 2000 and July 2002 (http://web.lexis-nexis.
com/universe/doclist?_m=182fd9ddb907aaba02d113aaafd04aca&wchp=
dGLbVzz-lSlzV&_md5=0f608d75f1961f5cf547659201d9bb41). Many
of them reported the challenges and successes that the Hmong Americans and the local American communities have encountered and con-
quered. A search on Infotrac (http://web7.infotrac.galegroup.com/itw/
infomark/0/1/1/purl=rc6_EAIM?sw_aep=csus_main) yielded 18 documents on Hmong Americans. Only a few of these documents were from
journal articles, and they were mainly from the disciplines of ethnic
studies, history, and economics. OCLC First Search database (http://
firstsearch.oclc.org/WebZ/FSQUERY?format=BI:next=html/records.
html:bad=html/records.html:numrecs=10:sessionid=sp02sw11-44519-
d4yhzpuu-xksize:entitypagenum=2:0:searchtype=basic) listed 17 articles from the *Sociological Abstract* about Hmong Americans. Only two
of these were published in social work journals.

Search for statistics from the National Institute of Health, National
Center on Minority Health and Health Disparities (http://ncmhd.nih.gov/);
National Institute of Mental Health (*http://www.nimh.nih.gov/home.htm*)
and the Special Programs Development Branch, Center for Mental
Health Services (*http://www.samhsa.gov/*) did not reveal any result on
the rate of Hmong or Southeast Asian persons classified as having disability including impairment as defined by the U.S Department of
Health and Human Services. A prominent leader of the Hmong communities in California estimated that about 20% of the Hmong Americans
are persons with disability.

DISABILITY AND HMONG SHAMANISM (UA NENG)

Barnes, Mercer, and Shakespeare (1999) viewed disability as a social
creation and the explanation of its changing character located in the social and economic structure and culture of the society in which it is
found. Wolfensberger (1980) contended that people with disabilities
are frequently labeled as deviant and assigned societal role expectations
based on stereotypes. Once defined as deviant, that person is expected
to play the deviant role (Barnes et al., 1999). Disability can sometimes
be perceived as a gift or test from god (Mackelprang & Salsgiver,

1999). Persons with disabilities may also be perceived as objects of pity (Wolfensberger, 1980).

Meaning, perception, and understanding about persons with disabilities are heavily influenced by society, politicians, and human service professionals. Disability has often been surrounded by unfavorable perceptions. It is the target of stereotyping rather than a reason for celebrating. Families of persons with disabilities normally do not receive the same view as Wolfensberger (1980) put it, "the primary cultural transmitter" (p. 137), where everyone should be valued and judged according to the group's cultural norms. When the primary cultural transmitter is absent, the families may be subjected to unfair judgment and criticism from people in the community. For example, a Hmong person with a disability may be perceived as not suitable to grow up in a family of his or her own or may be discouraged from attempting to start a family.

Vitebsky (1997) states that the word *shaman*, sometimes erroneously used interchangeably with sorcerer or medicine man, comes from the language of Evenk, a small group of Tungus-speaking hunters and reindeer herders in Siberia. Shaman can be seen as actors or performers because they share the arts of chanting, improvising, role-playing, and imagery, and they are capable of traveling to another world (Riches, 2001, p. 14). Harner (1982) described the shaman specifically as "a man or a woman who enters an altered stated of consciousness at will to contact and utilize an ordinary [sic] hidden in order to acquire power and to help other person" (p. 25).

Within the Hmong culture, there are *txiv neeb*-tsi neng (shaman) and *niam neeb*-nia neng (shawoman). Quincy (1995) suspects that shamanism might have been introduced to the Hmong by way of their past migration history from the Middle East to Southeast Asia; during this journey the Hmong might have been brought in contact with the Siberian shamans. Xiong (2001) wrote that Hmong shamanism is a traditional healing practice rather than a medicine man or a type of religion. There has been a misconception about Hmong shamanism in that it is often perceived as "the Hmong Religion." Xiong added that any Hmong shaman quickly points out this misrepresentation. Shamanism is a cultural concept and practice that is closely related to disability. While shaman/shawoman is always initiated through illness, their recovery begins their link to the healing spirits. From there they serve as healing intermediators and intervene in many difficulties encountered by Hmong Americans, including mental and physical illness and disabilities. Instead of being viewed as religious leaders, Hmong shaman/shawoman were more appropriately viewed within the Hmong community as elders, usually playing the role of community advocates and leaders.

Since the Hmong first arrived in the United States over a quarter century ago, healthcare agencies have usually prohibited a Hmong shaman/ shawoman from treating ill Hmong patients at hospital sites. Shamanism is viewed as irrelevant to Western modes of healthcare practice. Many shaman/shawoman were perceived as disabled, psychotic, or individuals suffering from some form of mental health condition. These incompatibilities have resulted in conflicts between the Hmong and health and human services professionals. In order to address this difference, several Hmong communities have formed coalitions to introduce the utilities of Hmong shamanism to doctors, nurses, and social workers. For example, with support from the Mayor's Office of Fresno, CA, and several city council members, a Hmong Shaman Committee was successful in legitimizing the use of a shaman/shawoman for Hmong patients in medical facilities there. The city lists and provides all Hmong shaman with a special identification card, which allows them to practice their healing. Shaman there can now go to the hospital and treat Hmong patients without restriction, except they must comply with the city's fire codes and animal rights (Executive Director P. Fang, personal communication, Lao Family Community, Inc., Fresno, CA, 1999).

SURVEY OF A SAMPLE OF HMONG AMERICANS

In order to develop a culturally competent approach to more effectively working with the Hmong populations, particularly on disability-related issues, the authors conducted an exploratory survey questionnaire with case scenarios targeting Hmong Americans in early 2002 in Northern California. The study aims to explore: (a) the targeted Hmong's knowledge about persons with disabilities; (b) their beliefs in regard to which Hmong subgroups have higher prevalence of disability; (c) their attitudes toward persons with disabilities; (d) their reactions toward specific case situations where the Hmong first seek help for their disability conditions; and (e) how well the Hmong continue to utilize informal networks within their community.

The authors recruited a snowball convenient sample of 100 Hmong Americans ages 18 to 65 who are able to read and write English and had expressed interest in this study. Out of the 100, three-page questionnaires distributed, respondents returned 83. Among them, four were discarded due to missing or incomplete data. At the end, the authors used 79 completed questionnaires for data analysis. Limitations in this study included: (a) only literate Hmongs were recruited as respondents; (b) a wide range of ages, from 18 to 65; and (c) the sample is not a representation of the Hmong Americans as an overall.

The survey questionnaire was written in mixed Hmong and English to fully convey the intention of the study. All English items were also back-translated into Hmong to ensure accuracy. The authors consulted three Hmong elders and asked them to comment on the cultural appropriateness and accuracy of all the questionnaire items. Due to their involvement in the development of the data collection instrument, these elders were not included as research subjects for the study.

The final 38-item survey questionnaire included 8 demographic information questions, 7 general questions about Hmong's knowledge about persons with disability, 10 questions on values and beliefs, and 13 case scenarios.

The term disability was deliberately not clearly defined for the study participants. Broad concepts, nonspecific to physical or psychological disability conditions, were used. In many situations, the authors employed terms in Hmong dialect that refer to disability such as *dig muag* (blind), *tej yam ua tsi yog yav tag los* (punishments from past life), or *vwm* (crazy) in the data collection instrument and the interviews. This nonspecific and open-definition approach allows the study to collect views on disability that are ethnographically and culturally appropriate to the Hmong respondents.

Study Participants

Of the 79 subjects, 46.8% (n = 37) were females and 53.2 % (n = 42) were males. The youngest ones were 18 and the oldest one was 65 (mean = 29.49, SD = 9.66). Length of residency in the United States averaged 20 (SD = 4.12) years and a range from 7 to 28 years. Seventeen (21.5%) of the respondents were born in the U.S., 7 (8.9%) were born at refugee camps in Thailand, and 50 (69.6%) were born in Laos. Among the Laotian-born respondents, 26 (47%) indicated they did not receive any form of education in Laos, 12 (22%) received between 1 to 8 years of schooling, and 7 (13%) received 9 or more years of schooling. All respondents have had an average of about 15 years of schooling in the United States. Eighteen (23%) had a master's degree or higher. Contrary to the primarily farming Hmong population with little formal education in their old rural Laos homeland, today one can easily find Hmong Americans who are well educated and professional.

As to their marital status, 32 (41%) of the respondents were single, 43 (55.1%) were married, and 3 (3.8%) were separated. More than a third of the respondents, 39.4% ($n = 26$) were assembly line workers; 18.2% ($n = 12$) were college students; 15.2% ($n = 10$) were human service providers; 9.1% ($n = 6$) were in business; 15% ($n = 10$) were employed at various professions or jobs such as teacher, nurse, engineer, interpreter, and food server; and 3% ($n = 1$) were unemployed.

Prevalence

Fifty respondents (64.9%) reported to have known someone who has a disability. Among them 86.8 % ($n = 46$) said that they either have a disabled family member or know a relative with a disability condition.

When asked about the prevalence of disability in the Hmong community, the majority of them (63.3%, $n = 51$) either believed that it was not prevalent (34.2%, $n = 27$) or had no knowledge (29.1%, $n = 23$) about disability among Hmong individuals. While 30.4% ($n = 24$) said it was moderately prevalent, only 6.3% ($n = 5$) viewed it as extensive.

One of the questions asked, "How much do they believe that disability is a major concern in the Hmong community?" revealed that overall, 37% ($n = 29$) believed that disability is a concern in the Hmong community.

The respondents were asked to rank the different age groups according to which they believed to have the highest numbers of persons with disabilities. Hmong participants ranked those aged 46 to 65 years as having the highest number of individuals with disability–51.9% ($n = 41$); the Hmong elderly ranked second with 24.1% ($n = 19$), and children (younger than 12 years of age) ranked third, 12.7% ($n = 10$). The rest of the percentages were distributed among Hmong aged 13 to 45 years. Respondents also believed that those born in Laos have had higher incidents of disabilities (47.4%). They were followed by those who were born in refugee camps (13.2%), and 31.6% said they did not know. This finding appears to be consistent with the general belief within the Hmong community that many Hmongs who were born in Laos, especially children born during and after the Vietnam War, were exposed to the war's weaponry chemicals. For example, even nearly three decades after the U.S. forces withdrew from Southeast Asia, the Communist Pathet Lao continued to bomb and used chemical and biological weapons against the Hmong. A current report by a U.S. Congressional Forum on Laos (*http://www.vientianetimes.com/Lao_forum/09182002_ us_congressional_forum_on_laos.html*) states that the Hmong continue to be chemically poisoned up to this very date. Even though the refugee-camp conditions were not pleasant, overall it was a haven for the Hmong refugees at the time. Starvation at the refugee camps was considered much less of a problem than the chemical weapons that they were exposed to in Laos. For this reason, the Hmong continue to believe that those born in Laos either then or now will continue to have a higher proportion of persons with disabilities.

BELIEFS REGARDING DISABILITY

A finding worth noting is the response to the question "Whether a disabled person should be loved and respected for just like any person without a disability?" A majority of 86.1% ($n = 68$) said they should not, 5.1% ($n = 4$) said they should, and 8.9% ($n = 7$) refused to answer. Based on the experience of one of the authors, who is ethnic Hmong and has been very involved in many Hmong Americans' cultural and social activities, this negative response contradicts the Hmong cultural traditions. The Hmong have a long tradition in which persons with disabilities were viewed and valued. According to Hmong customs, families who have a person with any type of disability usually maintain one of three philosophical opinions. First, the person may have been given by God to the family as a gifted child. Second, the family may be suffering from a spiritual punishment or wrongdoing from past life. Third, it is necessary to prevent the condition from extending to another generation, and the family must provide the disabled person with love, care, respect, and freedom from ridicule. It is also a Hmong tradition that when one sees a person with disabilities, no one should ridicule or stereotype against the person openly. The authors believe that the older Hmong generations still hold these three traditional cultural values toward persons with disabilities. The younger generation may, however, have a different opinion.

Another concept that is very different to the Hmong's traditional cultural values is specifically about disabled children. As stated above, Hmong traditional cultural values emphasize deep respect for the ones of less virtue, among them children who are born with physical conditions such as, for example, a missing limb. In Laos, the Hmong value children quite highly. Among the values they have toward children is their strong consensus that these children come to earth with three important symbols: (a) the babies bring with them a sign or messenger of past ancestors' misbehavior and wrongdoing, (b) they are spirited gifts from *pog suab yawg suab* [past ancestors], and (c) physical alteration is considered offensive to the spirits of past ancestors.

With these three beliefs in mind, many Hmong adults insist that Western medical procedures, therefore, should not be performed without consultation with a Hmong shaman/shawoman. However, 83.3% (*n* = 65) of the respondents in this study said they no longer hold this belief. Only 16.3% (*n* = 12) said they still strongly believe it. The authors stipulate that these contradictions occurred because the Hmong are still unclear on what really constitutes disabilities.

The study participants' responses toward children with disabilities are similar to those regarding a Hmong person (young or old) with disabilities. In Laos, disability usually refers to one of the three following specific conditions: (a) a birth defect, for example, a child born with a missing limb; (b) a *ruam* (mad-crazy) person; and (c) a severe bodily injury from the war. Other forms of physical or psychological conditions were mostly unknown to the Hmongs. The complicated classifications and definitions of disability in the United States and the different social and cultural systems add to the challenging transformation of beliefs toward disability by the increasingly diversified Hmong American populations.

RESPECT TOWARD HMONG SHAMAN

In regard to Hmong shamanism, 51.3% (*n* = 39) said they still somewhat respect Hmong shaman/shawoman, 11.8% (*n* = 9) said they still respecting the concept very highly, 25% (*n* = 19) said they no longer respect it, and 11.8% (*n* = 9) said they have no opinion. A large number of Hmong has been converted to the Christian faith after their arrival in the United States. Among the Hmong Christians in this study, one third (33.3%) of them said they are no longer interested in shamanism; the remaining 66.7% said they will continue to teach and educate others about shamanism. Based on the authors' knowledge about the Hmong community, they believe that at least one third of the Hmong still practice shamanism or use shaman as their healers.

CASE SCENARIOS

Finally, the authors gave the subjects 13 case situations regarding different types of potential physical and psychological disability conditions, including one nonspecific type question. They asked the subjects, "Who or where they would first seek help for each case scenario?" The authors identified the potential sources of helpers in the scenarios, including a shaman, an herbalist, family members, Hmong leaders, a medical doctor/physician, a mental health worker, a social worker, other spiritual healers, and others (to be specified by respondent). The general potential psychological question and four case scenarios that are most relevant to the authors' research objectives are reported here.

In an attempt to validate the authors' understanding about the Hmong and their modes of seeking help, one of the case scenarios states, "Who will you seek help for the person first when you notice that a 30-year-old Hmong man is having bad dreams?" Almost one third ($n = 24$, 31.6%) indicate talking to a shaman, 23.7% ($n = 18$) said a mental health worker, 15.8% ($n = 12$) indicate family members, and 11.8% ($n = 9$) indicate an herbalist. The remaining 8.1% of answers were split among Hmong leaders, social workers, and other spiritual healers.

Another case scenario said, "Whom will you talk to first, if a 30-year-old Hmong woman comes to you indicating that she is having bad dreams about the refugee camp experience?" Almost one third (31.6%) of the respondents said they would talk to a shaman, 23.7% would talk to a mental health worker, 15.8% would talk to a family member, 14.4% would talk to a Hmong leader or an herbalist, 3.9% would talk to a fortuneteller, and 1.3% ($n = 1$) would talk to a social worker.

The third case scenario analyzed in this study stated, "Who will you talk to first when a 68-year-old Hmong man who lost an eye during the Vietnam War comes to you and is asking you to find financial assistance?" Forty-six (60.5%) respondents said a social worker, eleven (14.5%) said family members, followed by nine (11.8%) who said a medical doctor. A small number (7.8%, $n = 6$) indicated they would seek financial assistance within the Hmong community, for example, shaman and Hmong leaders.

The nonspecific question stated, "Who will you seek help from first when you noticed that either your own child or a family member's child does not pay attention to you or his/her parents?" More than half (55.8%) indicated family members, 16.9% would seek help from Hmong leaders, 14.3% would seek help from a social worker, and only 2.6% would seek help from a medical doctor/physician. Even years after resettling in the United States, the Hmongs' primary source of dependency and support remains unchanged. This also confirmed what Lee (1993) found, that regardless of situation or need, the Hmong would seek help from family members and clan leaders first.

It is obvious that Hmong respondents differentiated the various natures of concerns for the scenarios and would seek help from appropriate professionals or leaders who have expertise for the areas of concern. Families continue to be the basic support and reference system. Shaman and shawoman are included in spiritually related issues, for example, dreams and ancestral signs. Their influence, however, is diminishing.

DISCUSSION

Yuen and Nakano-Matsumoto (1998) described how Asian American families deal with individual and family crises in regard to family and friends. Certain mental and social disabilities could be considered as a taboo "that is not recognized or discussed because of shame and stigma it brings to a family" (pp. 46-47). When the issue "reaches at a point where something has to be done, the family will first attempt to solve the problem within immediate or extended network to avoid embarrassment for oneself and the family. Seeking outside help may cause the family to feel shameful and only be done as a last resort" (p. 47).

Findings from this study on Hmong Americans reflect a rather similar pattern. The traditional internal support network, starting from families and relatives, is the primary source of support. Although traditional spiritual and cultural healing methods such as shaman are still being utilized, their usage has been going through certain modifications. Shamanism no longer plays the dominant role in healing among Hmong. Instead it is used in conjunction with or in support of the Western medicine and psychotherapeutic techniques.

A great degree of acculturation has taken place among Hmong Americans, particularly among the younger generations. Like many other new Americans, there are ongoing negotiations and transformation between the native culture and the ever-changing American culture.

Hmong people have their unique perceptions, beliefs, understanding, and respect of disability and persons with disabilities. These beliefs have been challenged and altered by modern American concepts and legal regulations of disability. Social workers who work with Hmong Americans on disability issues should be cognizant about the transformation and its implications for effective practice. When practicing with Hmong clients, it is the appreciation, dedication, knowledge, and skills in the coordination, inclusion, and utilization of the family, shaman, community leaders, Western medicine, and native folk beliefs that make a social worker culturally and professionally competent.

REFERENCES

Barnes, C., Mercer, G., & Shakespeare, T. (1999). *Exploring disability: A sociological introduction*. Malden, MA: Blackwell.

Hamilton-Merritt, J. (1993). *Tragic mountains: The Hmong, the Americans, and the secret war for Laos, 1942-1992*. Bloomington & Indianapolis: University Press.

Harner, M. (1982). *The way of the shaman: A guide to power and healing*. Toronto, Canada: Bantam Books.

Lee, S. C. (1993). *Stress, social support system, and psychological well-being of the refugee adults*. Unpublished doctoral dissertation, University of Washington, Seattle.

Mackelprang, R., & Salsgiver, R. (1999). *Disability: A diversity model approach in human service practice*. Pacific Grove, CA: Brooks/Cole.

Marinelli, R. P., & Dell Orto, A. E. (1999). *The psychological & social impact of disability*. (4th ed.). New York: Spring Publishing Co..

Mottin, J. (1980). *The history of the Hmong*. Bangkok, Thailand: Odeon.

Quincy, K. (1988). *Hmong: History of a people*. Cheney, WA: Eastern Washington University Press.

Riches, D. (2001). *Shamanism: The key to religion*. University Circle, Charlottesville, VA: University of St Andrews.

Vang, P. G. (2001). *2001 Hmong population and education in the United States and the world*. Wausau, WI: Lao Human Rights Council.

Vitebsky, P. (1997). What is a shaman? *Human Nature, 3*(97), 34-53.

Wolfensberger, W. (1980). The definition of normalization: Update, problems, disagreements and misunderstanding. In R. J. Flynn & K. E. Nitch (Eds.), *Normalization, social integration, and community service* (pp. 51-71). Baltimore: University Press.

Xiong, G. (2001). *Knowledge, utilization, and perceptions of shamanism and Western counseling or psychotherapy by the various Hmong subgenerational groups and religious beliefs*. Unpublished master's thesis, California State University, Fresno.

Yuen, F. K. O., & Nakano-Matsumoto, N. (1998). Effective substance abuse treatment for Asian American Adolescents. *Early Child Development and Care, 147*, 43-54.

Index

"Compulsory K-12 Special Education
    System," 69
"Disability: Social and Health Issues," 6
"Refrigerator parents," 12
"Supported Conversation," 52-53
"The Hmong Religion," 124
1981 International Year of Disabled
    Persons, 72

AAMR. *See* American Association on
    Mental Retardation (AAMR)
Acquiescence
    defined, 17
Ad Hoc Task Force on Social Work
    Education and Disability, 68
ADAPT, 10-11
Adaptation
    described, 18
AFP. *See* Alpha Feto Protein (AFP)
Alpha Feto Protein (AFP), 92
ALS. *See* Amyotrophic lateral sclerosis
    (ALS)
American Association on Mental
    Retardation (AAMR), 90
American Sign Language (ASL),
    26,28,31,36,41-42,43
Americans With Disabilities Act (ADA),
    10,13,16,20,68,89-90
Amyotrophic lateral sclerosis (ALS), 19
Analysis of Variance
    in MIDS, 76-77
Aphasia
    defined, 48
    described, 48

life participation approaches to, 47-64
    (*See also* Life Participation
    Approach to Aphasia (LPAA))
    as goal, 58-59
    availability of services in, 60
    environmental factors in, 60
    introduction to, 48-49
    life enhancement changes due to,
        59-60
    measures of success in, 59-60
    personal factors in, 60
    services for persons with, 59-60
    social approaches to
        in United States, 54-55
    stroke and, 48
    treatment of
        history of, 49-50
Aphasia Center of California, 53
Arthritis
    rheumatoid
        stigmatization of
        case example, 17
ASL. *See* American Sign Language
    (ASL)
Australia
    LPAA implementation in, 58
Autobiography
    in LPAA implementation
    in England, 57

Bahan, B., 25
Barnes, C., 123
Beck, I., 91
Behavior(s)
    human
        social environment effects on

in psychotherapy for deaf and
hard-of-hearing
persons, 41-42
norms of, 17-19
Bell, A.G., 12
Bernstein-Ellis, E., 53
Bettleheim, B., 12
Boles, L., 47,50,55,57,59
Byng, S., 57

California Welfare and Institutions code,
94
Canada
LPAA implementation in, 52-53
Carter administration, 67
CDPD. *See* Commission on Disability
and Persons with Disabilities
(CDPD)
Center on ASL Literacy, 27,28,29
Chapey, R., 50
Charity Organization Societies, 68
Cheung, J. C-k, 3,101
Children
deaf, 14
Chorionic villus sampling (CVS), 92
Cohen, C.B., 2,23
Commission on Disability
within Council of Social Work
Education, 43
Commission on Disability and Persons
with Disabilities (CDPD), 68
Communication
among deaf community
conflict related to, 11
in psychotherapy with deaf and
hard-of-hearing persons, 32-34
Communication Partners, 58
in LPAA implementation in United
States, 54
Communication rehabilitation

international perspectives on, 47-64
(*See also* Life Participation
Approach to Aphasia (LPAA))
Communist Pathet Lao, 127
Community
deaf, 25
communications methods among
conflict related to, 11
on deafness, 8
Community integration
defined, 103
of older people in Hong Kong with
disabilities, 101-119 (*See also*
Developmental disabilities, in
older people in Hong Kong,
community integration of)
Competence
cultural
described, 7-8
Corker, M., 38,41
Corporation on Disabilities and
Telecommunications, 9
Council of Social Work Education
Commission on Disability within, 43
Council on Social Work Education
(CSWE), 6,68
Cross cultural issues
in psychotherapy with deaf and
hard-of-hearing persons, 39-40
CSWE. *See* Council on Social Work
Education (CSWE)
Cultural competence
described, 7-8
Cultural knowledge
in deaf and hard-of-hearing persons,
30-32
Cultural sensitivity
described, 7-8
Culture
deaf, 25
defined, 7
disability (*See* Disability culture)

composition of, 9-10
disability as, 8-11
disability through lens of, 5-22 (*See
    also* Disability culture;
    Disability(ies), through lens of
    culture)
CVS. *See* Chorionic villus sampling
    (CVS)

DA. *See* Americans With Disabilities
    Act (ADA)
Damico, J., 50,54,58,59
Davis, G.A., 50
Deaf
    defined, 14
Deaf child, 14
Deaf community, 25
    communications methods among
        conflict related to, 11
    on deafness, 8
Deaf culture, 25
Deaf persons, 14
    psychotherapy with, 23-46
        bias with, 28-29
        communication in, 32-34
        cross cultural issues in, 39-40
        cultural knowledge in, 30-32
        data analysis procedures in, 29-30
        demographic information related
            to, 46t
        differential use of self in, 34-38
        ego/culturally syntonic
            interventions in, 38-39
        implications for social work
            education in, 41
        limitations of, 28-29
        methodology of
            development of, 27-30
        rationale for, 24
        social work policy in, 43
        social work practice in, 42-43
        study of, 26-27
Deafness
    deaf community on, 8

defined, 24-26
Department of Developmental Services,
    94
Department of Disability Services
        website
    of state of California, 94-95
Deutsche Lebenshilfe ev, 95
Developmental disabilities
    defined, 89
    in older people in Hong Kong
        community integration of, 101-119
        conceptual framework of,
            103-105,104f
        deficient social interaction in,
            113t,115
        discussion of, 115-117
        empowerment in, 112-115,
            113t,115t
        fair knowledge of community
            in, 108,109t
        from normalization to
            empowerment,
            115-117
        high level of perception of
            being accepted in
            community in, 110,
            111t
        inadequate *vs.* adequate,
            110-112
        lack of company in going out
            in, 107-108,109t
        less chance to have company
            in, 112-113,113t
        lesser use of social services in,
            113-114,113t
        levels of, 107-112,108t-111t
        limitations of, 117
        lower assertiveness in, 113t,
            114,115t
        moderate level of assertiveness
            in, 110,110t
        modest level of social
            interaction in, 107,
            108t

poor knowledge about,
113-114,113t
study of
methods in, 105-107,106t
results of, 107-112,108t-111t
Developmental Disabilities Assistance
and Bill of Rights Act of 1990,
89
dig muag, 126
Disability culture. *See also*
Disability(ies), through lens of
culture
advocacy groups for, 10-11
common history in, 12-13
composition of, 9-10
differences in, 10-11
economic concerns related to,
15-16,16t
future of, 19-20
mutual language in, 13-15
stigmatization of, 17
unity in, 10-11
Disability rights movement
in Japan, 69-70
in U.S., 67-68
Disability(ies)
among Hmong Americans
prevalence of, 127-128
as culture, 8-11
defined, 14,89-92,122
described, 14-15,124
early detection of, 92
economic concerns of people with,
15-16,16t
Hmong Americans views on, 121-132
(*See also* Hmong Americans,
disability views of)
Hmong shamanism and, 123-125
in utero detection of, 92
life with
norms of behavior in, 17-19
medical model of
described, 67
money for, 93
orientation after detection of, 92

persons with
attitudes toward
Analysis of Variance in, 76-77
correlation in study of, 76,77t
data analysis in study of,
74-81,75t-77t,78f-80f
demographics in study of,
74-75,75t,76t
discussion of study of, 81-83
exploratory study on involving
U.S. and Japanese
students, 65-85 (*See
also* Modified Issues
in Disabilities Scale
(MIDS))
findings of study of, 74-81,
75t-77t,78f-80f
instrumentation in study of,
73-74
item analyses in study of,
77-81,78f-80f
research methods in study of,
72-74
samples in study of, 72-73
t-tests in study of, 76,77t
services for (*See* Disability-related
services)
through lens of culture, 5-22 (*See also*
Disability culture)
introduction to, 6-8
time involved in, 93
Disability-related services
assessment of, 94
described, 94
early intervention in, 94-95
in U.S. and Germany
comparison between, 87-100
case example, 88-99
caution in, 88
introduction to, 87-88
medical services, 95-96
options in, 97-99
school services, 96-97
transition services, 97-99
Disabled in Action, 67

Drawing
  in LPAA implementation
    in England, 57-58
Duchan, J., 57

Early Start, 94
Economic concerns
  of people with disabilities, 15-16,16t
Education
  social work
    implications of
      in psychotherapy for deaf and
        hard-of-hearing
        persons, 41-43
    in Japan, 70-71
Education of All Handicapped
    Children's Act (EHA), 13
Ego/culturally syntonic interventions
  in psychotherapy with deaf and
    hard-of-hearing persons, 38-39
EHA. *See* Education of All Handicapped
    Children's Act (EHA)
Eingliederungshilfe, 98
Elderly
  developmental disabilities in
    in Hong Kong
      community integration of,
        101-119 (*See also*
        Developmental
        disabilities, in older
        people in Hong Kong,
        community
        integration of)
Elman, R., 53
Empowerment
  of older people in Hong Kong with
    developmental disabilities,
    112-115,113t,115t
Empowerment language, 16t
England
  LPAA implementation in, 57-58
Environment
  social
    human behavior effects of

  in psychotherapy for deaf and
    hard-of-hearing
    persons, 41-42
Environmental factors
  in LPAA, 60
Erzieungsgeld, 93
Erzieungsurlaub, 93
Eugenics era, 12
Eugenics movement, 12

Frank D. Lanterman Regional Center, 94
Fruehfoerderstellen, 95

Gailey, G., 51
Galludet University, 26,29,39
German Council of Education, 91
Germany
  disability-related services in, 87-100
    (*See also* Disability-related
    services, in U.S. and Germany,
    comparison between)
Gimp
  described, 18
Glickman, N., 30
Goddard, H., 12
Government Action Plan for Persons
    With Disabilities of 1995, 70
Group treatment
  in LPAA implementation in United
    States, 53-54

Handicapped
  defined, 15
  described, 115
Hard-of-hearing persons
  psychotherapy with, 23-46
    bias with, 28-29
    communication in, 32-34
    cross cultural issues in, 39-40
    cultural knowledge in, 30-32
    data analysis procedures in, 29-30

demographic information related
    to, 46t
differential use of self in, 34-38
ego/culturally syntonic
    interventions in, 38-39
implications for social work
    education in, 41
limitations of, 28-29
methodology of
    development of, 27-30
rationale for, 24
social work policy in, 43
social work practice in, 42-43
study of, 26-27
Harner, M., 124
Harris Poll, 15
Hawking, S., 19
Hayashi, R., 65
Heumann, J., 67,70
Hitler, A., 12
Hmong Americans
    described, 122
    disabilities among
        prevalence of, 127-128
    disability views of, 121-132
        case examples, 129-131
        discussion of, 131
        study of
            participants in, 126-127
    historical background of, 122
    news articles on, 123
    sample of
        survey of, 125-128
    U.S. population of, 122
Hmong shaman
    respect toward, 129
Hmong Shaman Committee, 125
Hmong shamanism, 124
    Hmong Americans and, 123-125
Hoffmeister, R., 25
Hong Kong
    developmental disabilities in older
        people in

community integration of, 101-119
    (*See also* Developmental
    disabilities, in older people in
    Hong Kong, community
    integration of)
Horte, 95
Human behavior
    social environment effects on
        in psychotherapy for deaf and
        hard-of-hearing persons, 41-42
Humane Society, 54

IDEA, 13,20. *See* Individuals with
    Disabilities Education Act
    (IDEA)
IEP. *See* Individualized education plan
    (IEP)
IFSP. *See* Individualized family support
    plan (IFSP)
Individualized education plan (IEP), 94
Individualized family support plan
    (IFSP), 94
Individuals with Disabilities Education
    Act (IDEA), 96-97
Individuals with Disabilities Education
    Act (IDEA) Amendments of
    1991, 94
Institute on Disability Culture, 9
International Classification of
    Impairments, Disability, and
    Handicap
    of WHO, 90-91
Inversion
    described, 18

JACSW. *See* Japanese Association of
    Certified Social Workers
    (JACSW)
Japan
    disability rights movement in, 69-70
Japan Society for Disability Studies, 70
Japanese Association of Certified Social
    Workers (JACSW), 71
Jerry Lewis telethon, 11

Kagan, A., 51,52,60
Kimura, M., 65
Kindergeld, 93
Kinderkrippen, 95
Knowledge
    cultural
        in deaf and hard-of-hearing
            persons, 30-32
Konig, A., 91
Kurzzeitbetreuung, 98

Lane, H., 25
Language
    empowerment, 16t
    mutual
        among disability culture, 13-15
Lathrop, D., 8
Lee, S.C., 3,121,130
Lewis, J., 11
Lewis, M., 47,55,59
LexisNexis, 123
Li, M. K-y, 3,101
Life enhancement changes
    LPAA and, 59-60
Life Participation Approach to Aphasia
        (LPAA), 47-64
    availability of services in, 60
    core values of, 51-52
    described, 48-49,51-52
    discussion of, 58-60
    implementation of
        in Australia, 58
        in Canada, 52-53
        in England, 57-58
        in United States
            communication partners in, 54
            group treatment, 53-54
            social approaches to, 54-55
            solution focused aphasia
                therapy, 55-57
        international, 52-58
    implications for social work, 60-61

life enhancement changes due to,
        59-60
Long-Term Care Insurance Act of 1997,
        71
Lou Gehrig's disease, 19
LPAA. *See* Life Participation Approach
        to Aphasia (LPAA)
Lyon, J., 54,58,59

Marshall, J., 57
Medical services
    disability-related, 95-96
Mental retardation
    defined, 90,91
Mercer, G., 123
MIDS. *See* Modified Issues in
        Disabilities Scale (MIDS)
Modified Issues in Disabilities Scale
        (MIDS), 2,65-85. *See also*
        Disability(ies), persons with,
        attitudes toward
    described, 66
    in exploratory study on attitudes
        toward persons with
        disabilities, 73-74
    rationale for, 71-72
    research questions related to, 71-72
Modified Issues in Disabilities Scale
        (MIDS) Total Score, 75-76

Nakano-Matsumoto, N., 131
National Association of Social Workers,
        71
National Center on Minority Health and
        Health Disparities, 123
National Institute of Health, 123
National Institute of Mental Health, 123
Ngan, R. M-h, 3,101
niam neeb-nia neng, 124
Nixon, R., Pres., 67
Normalization
    defined, 17
    described, 17-18
NOT DEAD YET, 11

OCLC First Search database, 123
Orgassa, U.C., 3,87

Parr, S., 57
Personal factors
   in LPAA, 60
Persons with disabilities
   attitudes toward
      exploratory study on
         among U.S. and Japanese social
            work students, 65-85
            (*See also*
            Disability(ies);
            Modified Issues in
            Disabilities Scale
            (MIDS))
Pinderhughes, E., 7
pog suab yawg suab, 129
Pound, C., 57,59,60
Program Plans and Service White
      Papers, 102
Psychotherapy
   with deaf and hard-of-hearing
         persons, 23-46 (*See also* Deaf
         persons, psychotherapy with;
         Hard-of-hearing persons,
         psychotherapy with)

Quincy, K., 124

Re-negotiation
   described, 18
Rehabilitation Act of 1973
   Section 504 of, 67
Respect
   toward Hmong shaman, 129
Retardation
   mental (*See* Mental retardation)
Rheumatoid arthritis
   stigmatization of
      case example, 17
Roberts, E., 67,70
Rolling Quads, 67

Roosevelt, F., Pres., 9
Sacchett, C., 57,59
Scheffe's post hoc test, 77
School services
   disability-related, 96-97
Self
   differential use of, 34-38
Sensitivity
   cultural
      described, 7-8
Settlement House Movement
   in 19th century, 68
SFAT. *See* Solution focused aphasia
      therapy (SFAT)
Shakespeare, T., 123
Shaman
   defined, 124
   Hmong
      respect toward, 129
Shamanism
   Hmong, 124
      Hmong Americans and, 123-125
Shapiro, J.P., 6
Simmons-Mackie, N., 50,54,58,59
Social environment
   human behavior effects of
      in psychotherapy for deaf and
         hard-of-hearing persons, 41-42
Social Security, 18
Social work
   LPAA and, 60-61
Social work education
   implications of
      in psychotherapy for deaf and
         hard-of-hearing persons, 41-43
   in Japan, 70-71
   in U.S.
      history of, 68-69
Social work policy
   in psychotherapy for deaf and
      hard-of-hearing persons, 43
Social work practice
   in psychotherapy for deaf and
      hard-of-hearing persons, 42-43

Social work students
   exploratory study on attitudes toward
      persons with disabilities by,
      65-85 (*See also* Disability(ies);
      Modified Issues in Disabilities
      Scale (MIDS))
Social Workers and Care Worker Act, 71
Solution focused aphasia therapy
   (SFAT), 59
Sozialamt, 95
Sozialpaedagogisches Zentrum, 95
Special needs
   described, 15
Special Programs Development Branch,
      Center for Mental Health
      Services, 123
Spinal Network, 20
Steven, P., Supreme Court Justice, 8
Stigma
   defined, 17
Stigmatization
   in disability culture, 17
   of rheumatoid arthritis
      case example, 17
Stroke
   aphasia due to, 48

Taoists, 1
tej yam ua tsi yog yav tag los, 126
*The Ragged Edge, Mouth, and New
      Mobility,* 14
Tower, K.T., 2,5
Transition services
   disability-related, 97-99
Tse, C., 1
Turner, K., 17
txiv neeb-tsi neng, 124

U.S. Census Bureau, 122
U.S. Congressional Forum on Laos,
   127-128
U.S. Department of Health and Human
      Services, 123

United Nations (UN), 2
United States (U.S.)
   disabilities rights movement in, 67-68
   disability-related services in, 87-100
      (*See also* Disability-related
      services, in U.S. and Germany,
      comparison between)
   LPAA implementation in, 53-57 (*See
      also* Life Participation
      Approach to Aphasia (LPAA),
      implementation of, in United
      States)
   social work education in
      history of, 68-69
University of California-Berkeley, 67

Vash, C.L., 8
Vietnam War, 122,130
Visiting Teacher Programs, 69
Vitebsky, P., 124
Vocational rehabilitation, 18
vwm, 126

Wade, C., 9
Walker, A., 116
Walker, C., 116
WHO. *See* World Health Organization
   (WHO)
Wilcox, M.J., 50
Wolfenberger, W., 123,124
World Health Organization (WHO),
   50,54,90-91
      International Classification of
         Impairments, Disability, and
         Handicap of, 90-91
Worrall, L., 58,59

Xiong, G., 124

Yuen, F.K.O., 1,3,121,131

BOOK ORDER FORM!

Order a copy of this book with this form or online at:
http://www.haworthpress.com/store/product.asp?sku=5047

International Perspectives on Disability Services
The Same But Different

____ in softbound at $22.95 (ISBN: 0-7890-2093-9)
____ in hardbound at $34.95 (ISBN: 0-7890-2092-0)

COST OF BOOKS _____

POSTAGE & HANDLING _____
US: $1.00 for first book & $1.50
for each additional book.
Outside US: $5.00 for first book
& $2.00 for each additional book.

SUBTOTAL _____
In Canada: add 7% GST. _____

STATE TAX _____
CA, IL, IN, MN, NY, OH & SD residents
please add appropriate local sales tax.

FINAL TOTAL _____
If paying in Canadian funds, convert
using the current exchange rate,
UNESCO coupons welcome.

❏ BILL ME LATER:
Bill-me option is good on US/Canada/
Mexico orders only; not good to jobbers,
wholesalers, or subscription agencies.

❏ Signature _____

❏ Payment Enclosed: $ _____

❏ PLEASE CHARGE TO MY CREDIT CARD:
❏ Visa ❏ MasterCard ❏ AmEx ❏ Discover
❏ Diner's Club ❏ Eurocard ❏ JCB

Account # _____

Exp Date _____

Signature _____
(Prices in US dollars and subject to change without notice.)

PLEASE PRINT ALL INFORMATION OR ATTACH YOUR BUSINESS CARD

Name

Address

City   State/Province   Zip/Postal Code

Country

Tel   Fax

E-Mail

May we use your e-mail address for confirmations and other types of information? ❏ Yes ❏ No We appreciate receiving
your e-mail address. Haworth would like to e-mail special discount offers to you, as a preferred customer.
We will never share, rent, or exchange your e-mail address. We regard such actions as an invasion of your privacy.

Order From Your **Local Bookstore** or Directly From
The Haworth Press, Inc. 10 Alice Street, Binghamton, New York 13904-1580 • USA
Call Our toll-free number (1-800-429-6784) / Outside US/Canada: (607) 722-5857
Fax: 1-800-895-0582 / Outside US/Canada: (607) 771-0012
E-mail your order to us: orders@haworthpress.com

For orders outside US and Canada, you may wish to order through your local
sales representative, distributor, or bookseller.
For information, see http://haworthpress.com/distributors

(Discounts are available for individual orders in US and Canada only, not booksellers/distributors.)

Please photocopy this form for your personal use.
www.HaworthPress.com

BOF04